Difference is Born on the Lips

'*Difference is Born on the Lips* is a brave, vulnerable, and beautiful book. Michael handles the toughest of subjects by weaving together personal and often difficult memories and life events with generous nuanced threads of magical, poetic prose. The pace of retelling is sublime; its incredible honesty a gift. A must read.'

Juno Roche, author of *Queer Sex* and *A Working-Class Family Ages Badly*

Difference is Born on the Lips

Reflections on Sexuality, Stigma and Society

MICHAEL HANDRICK

FL◆NT

For you

Thanks to James William Murray for the cover art: www.jameswilliammurray.com

First published 2022

FLINT is an imprint of The History Press
97 St George's Place, Cheltenham,
Gloucestershire, GL50 3QB
www.flintbooks.co.uk

British Library Cataloguing in Publication Data.
A catalogue record for this book is available from the British Library.

ISBN 978 0 7509 9902 1

Typesetting and origination by The History Press
Printed and bound in Great Britain by TJ Books Limited, Padstow, Cornwall.

Trees for LYfe

Omnia mutantur, nihil interit
Everything changes, nothing perishes

Ovid, *Metamorphoses*

Parts of this book may be triggering or upsetting. Please take your time. There are support services at the back of the book if you need them.

Prologue

What are our prologues? Who wrote them? Where did they begin?

On the council estate where I grew up? With the smell of pine and bluebells, and the stickiness of resin on palms in the woods nearby. Thorn-pricked fingers and blackberry-stained lips. Jam jar fishing in the river and fights in the alleys. The council estate where I snuck the 30 metres from my cousin's house to mine with the borrowed My Little Pony toy under my shirt. At school, where my identity didn't belong to me, it belonged to them. The ones who identified my sexuality, before I understood what sexuality was. The teachers and peers who bullied me because of where I grew up. The people who expected me to behave a certain way because of my working-class background. In the playground where I was forced to learn that some colours are dangerous. Where 'poof', 'faggot', 'batty', 'Billy Elliot' were chanted at me. Words hold power. Words shape. Difference is born on the lips.

The years I spent controlling my movements, my thoughts, my words, my accent; switching roles to be the masculine working-class boy I was supposed to be. Soon I could do it almost without thinking, automatically making an infinite number of adjustments, changes and corrections. I ensured that no imperfections, nothing that might be viewed as queer or effeminate, could leak out. I realigned unconsciously to behave as was expected, to the words that were written so deeply on my body as a child. From birth, I have had to shapeshift, alter my skin, change my movements, morph my tongue – unaware of how pretending to be someone else, of how lips pressed against my skin, would lead me down the path to abuse.

In bedrooms under tangled sheets. A place that had no direction, a room where compasses didn't work. Coiled together in the shadows, unseen by the eyes of others. Disentangle, retangle. Reliving and denying secrets we couldn't voice. Captives to our own yearning and chaos. The expectancy between us, clinging to each other; the expectancy that the night layered around us. That's all I knew: hidden touches and gasps under sheets and secrecy. Mornings cast with first light, sun-heated bodies as we drank each other. The evenings lit by unsteady moonlight, the windowpane fronded in frost, the iciness of the words that cracked in the night. The amulets on my necklace around index fingers, tugging me closer. Closer to harm.

The flick between love and hate, so easily slipping between the two. It felt dangerous to be me, to be with them, to be us. Away from the eyes and words of the people who would know right, put me in my place. Alone with them under loveless sheets. The cupid's bows pulled tight. Ready to fire. Shot with love, fired with hate, delivered with anger. Yet I did it anyway. There is power in words and voice. Love can impale. Abuse can impale. They strike from lips.

But no, that's not quite the beginning of it all.

There are many beginnings; it all depends on at what point we start to define ourselves. I wrote that many years ago, and it's something I come back to repeatedly. We think of life, memory and narrative as something linear: we are born, we grow, love and lose, and we die. There's a clear beginning and a clear end. But I've come to learn that's not the full story. Trust me, this isn't the beginning. Nor is it the end.

Once upon a time, I believed the abuse I went through was purely an isolated anomaly, an aberration in my story. It happened out of circumstance without any other influence or reason. Beginning. Middle. End. A glitch to forget and move on. Yet it ended up being the catalyst for me to examine my life and the influences in it that led me to those events. My exploration revealed that it wasn't the beginning or the ending. It was all part of a bigger chain of events and circumstances that I didn't know about until recently, but have shaped so many of my relationships, including the relationship with myself.

Only with time can you peel back the layers. Once there is nothing left to cover it, you see it for what it was.

Experiencing abuse so often isn't an isolated event with a clear beginning and end. It can be longitudinal and cumulative across a lifetime. There are years of other people, lovers, trauma and abuse – from childhood and early adulthood, and from before we were born – that weave together to lead us to that point. It's all part of the same and former existence. Nothing is destroyed, it simply changes. I've tried to follow the stepping stones back across time, space, memory and people. To discover who we will be in the future is to first recognise who we have been in the past and to understand how this affects us in the present. One cannot exist without the others.

After a good friend told me about a form of emotional attachment called trauma bonding, it allowed me to examine my life with a new lens. It gave me a new language to vocalise and actualise what has happened to me, both in the abuse I survived and the trauma I lived through in the past. That new lexicon stitched itself to my bones, my skin, my tongue. All the echoes of the former lives and bodies I have had to live, sewn up together. Frankenstein's new creation. It gave me a chance to live anew.

My efforts to understand trauma bonding and abuse, why it happens and how I could break the cycle, awakened forgotten and dormant memories and events. I can now see how they contributed to me ending up experiencing abuse. Coming out the other side of a cycle of abuse was a critical point that forced me to understand my past in the hope of creating a new beginning. It allowed me to understand that the beginning of those relationships started many years before, even before I was alive.

I've often wanted to purge my brain of events, and people, and actions and words. Of the abuse I've suffered from men, of the abuse from growing up gay and working class, of the stigma and expectations put on me by society because of my identities. These experiences are written across, on, and in my body. They regenerate even as the skin sheds and grows anew, when my body feels a new one against it, when I am under half-empty sheets thinking of the streets I ran down barefoot as a child, the life I could have had if everything had been different. They wait to unfold and bloom. The memories of the past become the memories of the future. I'd love a way to isolate those memories, separate them like isotopes, graft one memory onto another and create a new element. One without the fear, one without the pain, one without the words.

Memories are never true. We adapt, we falsify, we destroy memory. They are in constant motion, adjusting to agendas or in flux with other memories, with other people's memories. Beginnings and endings collide against one another. Two stories crashing together. We don't get to decide which has more force and which will prevail, or which is actually true. Memory is a record of our voice, our consciousness and the echoes that ping back and forth, calling to each other, but never with quite the same answer.

It's a revelation of the then in the now. The folding and unfolding of those moments across time and in this time. I've moved through time and memory and dream, what has become myth, what is truth. I navigated through beginnings and endings, unpicking where one thing crashed into another, where time and memory have merged, to try to understand how it all happened. Trying to understand my history, how each memory and each life spun up into something new. Nothing is linear. Time likes to rose tint. We cut out what hurts. Can we trust ourselves? Can we trust what we remember to be true, or are we coerced to doubt ourselves by time, other people and society? History is always written by the winner.

If my current or future self travelled back in time to warn my former self about them and what was to come, would it have made me wiser? Would I have listened? Would it have changed the trajectory of my story? No, because the genesis of my story would have been unaltered, the wheels were in motion before they arrived. The foundations had already been laid long before my own story had begun, and my childhood was the first layer of brickwork. They just built up from there. If it wasn't them, it would have been someone else waiting in the shadows to entice me with words, sighs and fingers running across my back. The voice I thought was telling me I was finally home was a warning from my future self. By the time the screams had passed through time, it would have been nothing but an extra beat against my heart mistaken for the pangs of desire and love.

Nothing is destroyed: basic chemistry. Whether this is breaking carbon bonds or the chemistry of love. Every instance of our lives is made up of former existences, past skins, past lovers, past stories. While I wish to forget what has happened, deny what they did or remain in denial, it all influences me in the past and in the now and in the future. It remains as part of my existence – tightly coiled to my DNA. The past can't be shifted, we can only learn to carry it differently and understand it to break cycles. We can write about it to make others aware.

For gay men, other people have been busy writing our prologues long before we are born. For a long time, I believed the abuse I went through was bad luck, the result of some random incidents, and not connected to the main narrative of my life. It was when I sat down and dissected what had happened to me that I began to understand and piece together the various threads that led me to that point. What I realised was that this was not something individual to me where I fell into a series of unfortunate events. It wasn't my prologue – it had all been long in the making without me knowing, by other people, other forces.

The more I researched, the more it became apparent that this is a systemic issue that relates to all gay men from the moment we are born. It's a symptom of being somehow outside of what in 2003 Lisa Duggan called the 'homonormative', where wider society and the dominant voices within it impose 'normal' heterosexual ideals and cultural practices onto LGBTQ+ people. They commend those who 'fit' into this selective microcosm of a diverse and multifaceted community. Being somehow outside of the homonormative adds detail to the prologues of working-class men, Black men, fat men, Asian men, religious men, disabled men, people living with HIV, people who identify with the letters beyond the first two of LGBTQIA. My story is only one example of how the personal and systemic are intertwined, and there are so many other possible entanglements.

So much of the abuse gay men go through is left unacknowledged, unknown or swept back into the closet. The multiple rapes and murders committed by Stephen Port between 2014 and 2015 were overlooked by chronic institutionalised homophobia. The country erupted in horror and outrage, in 2020, after Reynhard Sinaga was jailed for drugging and raping 48 men in Manchester. But the outrage over these big headlines doesn't fix the everyday suffering. It doesn't fix the daily hate crimes, the accrued discrimination across a queer person's life that leaves its mark, which so often goes unseen by society. There is so much more unknown by the wider public. The abuse gay men are victims of, and the mental consequences of this, amount to a largely unspoken epidemic, even within the gay community.

In adulthood we continue to live with the private battle of growing up as gay. There is a lack of reporting on male abuse and its consequences: untold mental health problems, addiction, self-destruction and suicide. In 2010, Human Rights Campaign reported that 26 per cent of gay men have experienced rape, physical violence, or stalking by a partner.[1] According to a 2012 Stonewall report, 49 per cent of gay and bisexual men suffered from domestic abuse.[2] Half of respondents to a 2018 Stonewall survey experienced depression, and one in eight 18–24-year-olds had attempted to take their lives.[3] The years pass by and the reports keep showing the same cycle of pain.

These figures could be higher: some people don't or can't report their abuse; they might not have the words to describe it, they might be too scared, they might not be ready to voice it. This endemic stems from wider institutional and cultural issues. For instance, the devastating impact of Section 28 implemented by a Conservative government in 1988, which banned teaching young people about LGBTQ+ issues until 2003. There was no offence for male rape until 1994, and only in 2004 was same-sex domestic abuse included in the Domestic Violence, Crime and Victims Act. It's resulted in our childhoods being stolen from us. We were taught that we weren't normal by our peers, our family, teachers or neighbours, or strangers who felt entitled to tell us in the street. We weren't taught the power of 'no'. We weren't taught that men can be abused, and, after all, men shouldn't express emotion and simply need to 'man up'. So many of us suffocate ourselves and suffer in silence because our words have been stolen, we aren't believed, and we didn't know this could happen because we'd never been taught about it.

What is it that's so rotten in our society that, despite our civil rights, we are still maligned and savaged as a community? I needed to understand why I have battled so many mental health issues. Why I had gone through abuse by men without even knowing it could happen. Without even realising it was happening to me.

Despite Section 28 having been revoked in 2003, LGBTQ+ education is still lacking and we are still not teaching young people – queer and straight – what they need to have healthy relationships with themselves and others, what is acceptable and not. Young people lack safe spaces to explore what it means to be gay. Many gay men don't know they can be raped. Many will knowingly or unknowingly replicate the abuse they have suffered. Despite gaining equal rights, including same-sex marriage, the discrimination and mental health issues the queer community suffer are rising, especially for those beyond the homonormative.

Despite the horrifying figures that show how the gay community is suffering, there is little movement to address this from central government. Successive Conservative governments led by David Cameron, Theresa May and Boris Johnson stalled on passing laws to ban conversion therapy, which equates to torture, and announced in March 2022 that it would proceed with the ban but without including our trans siblings. Protections for our trans siblings are slim and yet still apparently a matter of debate, with waves of campaigns to remove the few rights trans people do have. Laws matter. Education matters. Awareness matters. They are the difference between life and death. Someone being bullied or killed. Someone being free. It can mean affecting and scarring a person for the rest of their lives.

As queer people, our lives are irrevocably tied to the heterosexual: the cis, heterosexual legislators voting against civil rights, the institutionalised queerphobic judiciary and police force who don't believe a report of abuse or rape, the heterosexual family and friends who don't accept us for who we are. We are born into life with an inheritance, an inheritance that is formed before conception. Society and structures are geared up to heterosexual privilege and systemic queer oppression. No matter how hard we try, no matter how some of us might try and pretend otherwise, we are defined by that inheritance.

Cultural historian José Esteban Muñoz states that in the 'attempts to document a queer past, there is often a gatekeeper, representing a straight present'.[4] How do we record the queer past when it is dominated and constricted by the heterosexual? How do I vocalise it without the correct language? How do we document abuse between people of the same gender when there is so little precedent, when this has only legally been a concept for a few decades? How do we as queer people scrutinise our pasts and experience when, until about fifty years ago, we were illegal? How do we understand the queer experience in totality across all intersections when 'until recent decades very few lesbians or gay men outside of the upper (middle) classes left written records of their queer lives'?[5]

When for so long we've been forced to live in shadows and secrecy, when the gay working-class voice is a whisper trapped in the mind, conditioned to believe we will achieve nothing and have no worth. Conditioned to believe we can't be gay. When we have been tied down and gagged. When we have been given no voice, or our voices fall on ears that don't wish to listen.

My story comes from that place. I've sought to understand how our laws, the media, education, culture, have all created an environment from our childhood that primes gay men to suffer from abuse and mental health issues. An environment where abuse and trauma crept into my relationships without my even knowing it or realising it. Many people, even friends and family, don't realise that once a gay person has stepped out of the proverbial closet, our lives are not suddenly resolved and absolved from the trauma we have suffered. It is the very beginning of a process, in which we must find our true selves and reckon with what has happened. It is a process of shedding an identity we have mimicked our whole lives and trying to figure out who we are in this gay new world.

Our prologues were written by other people. We have been given narratives, structures and stories that don't belong to us, like characters pushed around in a plot by an author. I could have stood by and not said a word, ignored it happening, turned a blind eye and accepted that I was okay, that the world was okay. Accepted the story given to me by other people. But I needed to rewrite the narratives given to us by society or other people. We need these stories to help others understand, to help ourselves understand. There comes a point when we need to say 'no more' and call things out for what they are. My story could have slipped silently into history. But my brothers and sisters who fought for the rights we have today didn't achieve that by being meek. Long gone is the point where I could remain silent and grateful that I'd been given some equal rights. It's time to get loud. It's time to shout.

This is my story, and I hope it can also speak to our wider story, not just gay men but all queer people, to reclaim what was taken from us, to tell of the childhoods that were taken from us, to tell of the lives we weren't allowed to live. This book tries to understand what has created the epidemic of abuse and cyclical trauma within the gay community. It's an attempt to demonstrate how we overcome what has happened in the past, to stop the pain of the present and give us the future we deserve.

At the end of every story there is a full stop that allows us to close it and start another afresh. A new narrative to unfold. A new language to be spoken. A new chapter to begin. My nan always said, 'Speak the truth.' So here I am, as she told me, speaking the truth. I told you there were many beginnings and many endings, so let us begin.

Chapter One

The clock had struck twelve, the dings drowned out by the screams, the singing, the laughing. Twelve dancing princesses, all light and air. Twelve brothers, ravens in the night. A wolf in the dark. Tick, tick, tick. Time's running out. Time lost, must find time. When did we start mining for time? Follow the path, get home safe. Don't stray, quick. The final strike. Time has run out; the magic has run out. The dancing stopped; masks pulled off. We had our time, and time ran out. It's fleeting like passion.

I'd been at a fairy tale performance night with a best friend. We stepped from the safety of the club to the street. Shadows and men circled around us. The laughter at me. *Look at that queer. Wearing a crown. Fucking faggot.* The pounding of my chest, the throbbing of my heart in my mouth. My friend swearing at them. Their words, taunts lingering in the dark.

The slap of my card against the card reader. Splashes of beer, vodka, syrupy alcopops on my chest. The dark eyes edged in liner, the beard, his lips on mine. Watch out for the big bad wolf. Awoken with a kiss. He tasted like rum. The bite of my lip. The drops of blood. *The better to eat you with!* Numbers exchanged. Lust traded. Names not swapped. No glass slippers for me to pick up. Keep hunting for the fairy tale ending. My friend's hug and warmth in the rain outside the station. Slumping against the handrail on the Tube. The tears I didn't feel. The darkness.

I stared at the ceiling stitching together the fragments of the night. The duvet coiled around me; the pillows tossed to the floor during alcohol-soaked dreams. The undrawn blinds framed a broken grey sky. Fern fronds of ice had spiralled across the window, the floor mossed with tobacco from the pouch that must have fallen from my pocket. The red velvet coat I wore that night was strewn limply on the floor, figureless and waiting to be hung up in the cupboard along with my other dead selves. The crown next to it, broken. I had no idea what time or how I'd got home. I wanted to black out and forget. I achieved it every time I went out. Blocked out any residual remains of the past. Tried to burn the memories from my brain, eradicate the presence of the abuse I'd gone through in my body. So, I kept feeding that wavering darkness inside that was insatiable. Hoping the more I fed it, the more it would want, until I had consumed and drunk and fucked enough for it to overwhelm me. The summer was the perfect excuse to cover it up. The picnics and post-work drinks in the sun-baked parks with friends and colleagues, which would slide into pubs or bars or clubs. Another one, just one more, keep going. I knew my limit and I'd demolish it until the blackness crept across my vision and I'd wake up fully clothed on the bed trying to hide from the prying light.

I didn't care because it worked for a while. It stopped me thinking, it stopped me remembering. I kept running and kept moving and kept partying and kept myself busy because to stop would have meant really collapsing, beyond just collapsing to sleep. It would have given me the time and space to acknowledge everything properly. Not that I didn't think about them – they consumed my thoughts – but I didn't want to properly process it all and understand what they had done to me. I didn't want to feel anymore. I welcomed emptiness.

I wondered why I hadn't burned out, as winter arrived and the cold turned the permanent pool on the rooftop outside my window into a frosty mirror. I thought in the last strains of the summer heat, in the abating warm winds and blazing afternoons that I would have reached my zenith. I'd blazed my way through those months of crisp mornings, finding myself under crisp sheets, next to drying, crisp bodies that had been moist and sticky in the night.

I created fictions of myself underneath sheets, as love and guilt crusted on my hands and lips. I didn't move to pull on clothes to see them out, to hug them goodbye as if this were the beginning of something more. I couldn't even be bothered to seal the story shut with a kiss. I'd pull the half-empty sheets over my head to sleep off those fleeting exchanges of lust. It'd take longer to wash out the remains of our night than it would for me to forget about them. Is disgust and arousal the true recipe for love? How can both things be fed by the same root?

Yet summer had faded and I hadn't stopped. I hadn't stopped running. My mouth was dry, my throat hoarse from the chain smoking. The mornings were darker, and my mind darker and my thoughts darker. I groaned under the duvet. My eyes burned as I stared at the miniscule meshes of the woven fabric, longing for more sleep. The sheets served as a screen with faces projecting in front of me. The scenes of abuse and hate wrapped up in love and lust flickered at the back of my eyes, spinning in my mind, which kept me awake every night. Jolting awake, panting, the room empty yet filled with their words.

My phone vibrated. I took a deep breath and exhaled slowly before touching the home button to see who it was. It'd become one of my many new habits even though I knew it would be a friend or family. Yet every time my phone screen glowed it illuminated the fear of darker messages in me. I stretched my hand out from under the sheets and squinted at the screen.

It was already deep into the afternoon and I hadn't even moved properly. My friends from university were asking if we were still getting together that evening and where we'd be meeting. This was the distraction and company I craved. *Southbank?* I sent and smiled. The same place we had met for seven years. It was where we gathered at night during university to workshop our writing, drink and gossip. We always floated new places to try out, new bars, new pubs, new restaurants, but we inevitably always found our way back to the Southbank. It felt unnatural to imagine seeing them in a different London location. The workshopping had slowly faded out, but the habit was still there, the friendships remained.

I pulled myself up and rested my head against the headboard, the blood draining down my body. I stared at the ceiling, the dull thud of my pulse in my temples vibrated around my skull and settled behind my eyes. There was a knock on my door and I called out for them to come in.

My housemate rested against the doorframe. 'Another late one?'

'I'm assuming so.' I winced up at her and pulled the sheets up past my nose.

'Get showered, eat some beige food. Around for dinner?'

'No, out again later. Sorry.'

She laughed and shook her head at me. I pulled myself out of bed, opened the window and looked out across east London. Anish Kapoor's twisted sculpture a red pretzel on the horizon, the cranes lifting and turning. I turned on the shower and left it running to heat up. I stared at my face in the mirror until it steamed up.

There were still flecks of gold on my face and across my body from the night before. The gold my housemate had painted on my eyelids had dripped down my face like the crown I'd worn had melted onto my flesh, some golden golem an alchemist had sculpted and welded from the depths of their imagination. The skin under my eyes was mottled with violet and yellow like blossom in the spring, the glamour long worn off. I was never going to be that prince, the one with the fairy tale ending all tied up nicely in a bow. I was just a boy playing prince, being silly in make-up. *Mirror, mirror on the wall, who is the gayest of them all?*

There's a reason why I've always loved dressing up: it lets me become someone else, live a different story. I can create my own narrative and become a different person. Leave my body in the closet and slip into a new one. Escape from the person I was forced to be so I could find the true me, even just for a night. If I kept throwing on new characters, maybe after a while one would fit. You never get used to not feeling like you don't belong in your body, in the world. I am my own Bluebeard, locking up my former selves in the cupboard.

I thought of the guys from the night before, taunting me, calling me names just like when I was a kid. As if I needed to be reminded that I was different. Yet those words, so old and familiar like a childhood friend, still wielded the ability to cut in two. I'd become what those kids on the estate always said I was. *Fucking faggot.* I'd embraced it, accepted it, learned about it. But something about those words and threats, no matter how old I became, how much pride I'd learned for who I am, made me regress. I thought of the love I'd found and the fear that had been left in its place. How we're promised the former but never warned about the latter. I thought how tired I was of the weight inside me, of constantly pulling myself up every day and smiling like what we had – like I – was fine.

The tiredness from my eyes will at some point blow away, the purples and yellows disappearing in the first summer wind. What scared me the most was not knowing what damage had been done inside, unseen, and whether or not it would ever heal. Not knowing what all the years of hurt and abuse and pain had done to me. Trauma to the body is trauma to the mind that resurfaces once more as trauma to the body. The moments are still there, patterned in my body, on my flesh, each leaving their own stamp. A trail for me to follow if only I could decipher what it all meant.

Under the shower, I slumped against the tiles, my skin puckering from the heat. Constantly trying to shower them, him, off me. Marks and stains that just won't scrub off. Trying to clean away the rot that I felt inside. Wash away the tears, my cries drowned out by the shower's spray. I dug my nails into my skin to stop myself from screaming.

There were all these chunks and fragments and pieces and shards that I'd taped and glued and bandaged and tried to slot together. But some had crumbled, been lost, obliterated, or no longer fit. I kept scrambling to try to keep them together, making sure they weren't lost, just trying to hold them all together. Looking down at my arms cradling the pieces of me, all the times in life that I'd been broken and fixed and broken and put back together again and broken again, and the thought remained fixed in my mind that I didn't want to hold it all together anymore. The weight was too much, the expectation too much, my arms were shredded from the pieces. What happens when you feel like life has broken up with you?

Wrapped in my towel, I sat on the edge of my bed, convincing myself to get changed and leave even though I just wanted to stay home. It was at least the thirtieth bed I had slept in during my twenties. The suitcases with split zips from repeated overstuffing were still half unpacked from the latest move. Boxes still sealed shut. There was the picture of me and my cousin, Steph, at Brighton Pride on the windowsill, which was always the first to be unpacked; the lacrosse stick leaning in the corner I hadn't touched in eleven years; the plastic wallet filled with ticket stubs, exhibition and theatre brochures; stacks of books that needed to be slotted away.

I threw on some clothes, a scarf around my neck and went into the living room to grab my backpack. The hum of Kingsland Road outside the window filled the room: the buses, the laughter and shouts of people heading into Dalston, the music filtering out from the bars. The background noise was a comfort when my housemates were out. I switched off the floor and desk lamps that littered the room. I'd only been here a short time, but for the first time in a long time I could find moments of happiness. The Bonfire Night we had indoors grilling barbecue food and making mulled wine as it was too wet to go on the rooftop. The dinners where we all laughed at the fish-shaped water jug that glugged when you poured a glass. My best friends were a ten-minute walk away. There were people nearby in case I needed them if the words and the fear came back.

I pulled open the door and paused. Breathing. Waiting. Convincing myself to breach the threshold and that it'd be safe for me to go outside. An old habit that wasn't going. I didn't need to peer outside the door. I didn't need to do my breathing exercises to decrease my heart rate. I didn't need to chain smoke before getting on the Tube. I was safe here.

I put on my headphones and pulled out a book to distract my thoughts, keep my eyes focused to stop myself checking who was coming on, who was sitting behind me. Seeing words and phrases that were used against me, my chest would tighten. Just letters strung together to form a word, but those words have transformed into something bigger than that, more powerful and terrifying in my mind than I ever thought words could be. Knowing if I looked into the window, the bags under my eyes would be empty sockets in the reflection, absorbing the tears into nothingness.

The pages quivered in the spine as my leg shook, my heel bashing the floor. Every vibration from my phone in my pocket made me hold my breath. Were the streams of message notifications another cycle of missing me, hating me, blaming me, loving me? Every moment, every interaction was retraining myself that it had all finally stopped. I pushed the stop button.

I wrapped my scarf around my neck and my arms around my body as I walked over the bridge to the Southbank. To this day, every time I'm on that bridge I stop, even for a minute, to look up at Westminster. The white and red and blue and pink of London's lights, like fairies gently drowning in the black silky Thames. The drama of the ancient smashing into the ultramodern. Every time I looked out, I saw the millions of people out there dancing and crying and singing and dining from all over the world; I reminded myself that I made it here. From the council estate out in the countryside, I'd made it in London.

I weaved in and out between the crowds, big paper bags stuffed with Christmas gifts, scarves caught in the wind, the crackle of chestnuts being roasted. No matter the season, ice or blaze, the Southbank has always been one of my favourite spots. The string lights slinked between lamp posts, skateboarders and theatregoers raving or moaning about what they'd just seen at the National. The Christmas stalls were up, bratwurst crisping, the painted trinkets, the sizzle of churros being fried, sugar crystallising on lips.

My friends were already sitting outside the pub, huddled up against the cold. I hugged them both and slotted down under the patio heater with my drink.

'How are you?' A question that is so quotidian – so ordinary – so reflexive. But it was asked with so much genuine interest and concern that it took me off guard. I wanted to reply, 'I'm really not okay', but I'd been trained not to. Must look like I'm fine, carrying on, holding my head up. Be strong like the good boy I was supposed to be.

'Yeah, I'm okay, thanks.' I kept staring down, focusing on rolling the tobacco in the Rizla as I knew if I made eye contact with either of them in that moment I'd break. We didn't see each other every week, or even every month, but when we did those were the times when I headed home feeling warm and safe. Their laughter always took me back to university where we'd sit scribbling down stories to our tutors' prompts. The evenings spent together sitting on the floor in the Southbank Centre by the windows, the Thames a dark ribbon outside, as we gave each other feedback on our work. We talked about books, work, life, debating as we always did. We moved on to our 'love lives', of loves long gone.

'I've actually been doing some reading about something called trauma bonding.' One of my friends had recently been processing and researching a previous traumatic relationship to understand what had happened and why.

'What's that?' I asked.

'It's basically an act of abuse, countered by love or affection, trapping the abused person. The combination of a cycle of fear and reward creates intense emotional highs and lows that the abused person becomes reliant on. The abuser says they have displeased them, that they need to be punished, and in return the abused person then acts in a way to get back their affection and love, to prove that they are still worthy of the abuser. What they don't realise is that it's the abuser manipulating the whole thing to make them submissive to them.'

I kept drinking, looking out at the Thames and the people walking past. Some holding hands, some holding each other, others laughing. The times I'd been kissed in the mornings, begged to stay, told I was needed, told I was loved. Then it was my fault. I wasn't good enough. I'd ruined everything. Insulting me, blaming me, holding me. Different faces, same techniques, same cycles. I breathed in deeply, looking at the stars thrashing in the river, gasping for air. I lit another cigarette, wiping the tobacco remains off the bench, already starting to glisten with frost.

'So, basically, a cycle of abuse followed by love or affection? You become trapped?'

'In essence, yes. Bonded, trapped – all semantics.'

'Sounds about right,' I laughed, the only response I could give without crying. The times I'd kept what I'd been going through, what people had put me through from my friends and family. The times I'd said I was fine, it was fine. The horrifying feeling of loneliness and fear even though there was someone next to me in bed. Their body half illuminated by the moonlight, half in darkness. The many times I tried to leave, to escape, to block, to run but never quite able to do so. Nothing that was done to me, nothing that was said, nothing anyone else said, nothing I said to myself seemed enough.

I always justified it: too much alcohol, pride was hurt, a bad day. It's fine. Never normally like that. It was an anomaly. I promise I won't go back again. Just like passion and love; lies jump quickly from the lips to protect or cover shame and fear. I knew something wasn't healthy. I didn't realise it had been abusive. It felt normal. I'd created some myth in my mind, a space where a prince dwelled in my imagination. We story tell, fabricate, to self-preserve. Something was tethered, *bonded,* in those relationships and nothing seemed to sever it.

I unclamped my teeth and unfurled my hands from the fists they'd been in. The little, red 'C' marks fading quickly from my palm as if they'd never been there. It was the same if anyone looked at me; nothing had happened because they couldn't see any marks on my skin.

My friend had been through similar experiences, and even when she spoke about what had happened to her, I couldn't see or understand that I was following the same path. It wasn't possible. For some reason my mind forced me to unknow the reality of what was happening and what I was being bonded to. The world had conditioned me to not know this could happen to me. It took me months to tell them both what was happening. It was my friends who told me that what I had been going through was abusive. Even then I didn't believe that's what it was. It wasn't abusive, it couldn't be.

'I suppose it explains why I always went back.' I swigged from the pint glass, averting my eyes from them. Not wanting to be seen, embarrassed that it had happened. That I hadn't been able to recognise what had happened to me.

'Yeah, it sort of explains why so many people say, "Why don't you just leave?" Because there's something psychological going on where you become attached and dependent on the person,' my friend added. I nodded in agreement, thinking about the cases you hear on TV or in films or books where you often think, *If it's so bad, they should just leave.* But these stories had always been about men and women; I'd never seen anything that depicted same-gender abuse.

We kept talking about life, work, books, films until it was late and the dregs in the glasses remained untouched and there was no desire for the glasses to be filled. As the night grew colder and darker, I felt the same inside. The news, the night, the year. Not knowing what to do, how to handle it, what this meant for me. My friend lived out of town and had to catch the train. We booked in another date to meet up. *Southbank?* We hugged goodbye, and I lingered longer than I normally would.

'We're going to be okay,' she whispered. I watched them cross Blackfriars Bridge, grateful to have friends in my life who were there to support and look out for me. At the bus stop, I hugged myself, realising just how cold it was standing there alone in the dark, repeating to myself over and over that it would be okay.

Once on the bus, I looked up trauma bonding. What I read made more and more sense. How trauma bonding is more likely to occur when the person has been through some kind of abuse or trauma in their past – in a sense, making them more susceptible because they've been through something similar before. A clarity, a movement in my bones, folding over nerves, redirecting thought and movement. Something inside began to change. Memories and people and faces and events reaching out to each other, jigsaw pieces that could finally slot together. New thought patterns began to stitch and weave and graft to one another, sewn up from the inside.

As I shuttled through the night on the bus, I whispered into the silence and darkness where memory is archived. Deep in my body, in the echoes of dreams, in the sighs and cries and laughter, in the unvoiced words, I began to sift and shift through the years of my life to piece it all together.

Where did it all begin?

I closed the door behind me, it was dark and warm and empty inside. I switched on all the floor lamps in the living room for when my housemates got back. The fish jug stood proud on the kitchen table. I hung up my jacket, wiped off the tear dust and sat down on the edge of the bed looking at the boxes in the corner of the room.

I pulled off the tape on one box and inside was another one, a matryoshka doll of memories, where I sealed away the trail of lost love: letters, tickets, receipts, books, kisses in the rain, cuddles in the morning as spring's light spied on us, the twisting of events and emotions, being locked outside at night in the rain. A mausoleum to love and abuse. What was inside was supposed to be ephemera but had become relics. Those memories stored away like in glass boxes in a museum. I eulogised the past as if the present didn't exist, as if I had never made it out of the past. Why does no one ever think about what happens to the love left behind? Love is not an equation, it's not a myth, it can consume. We fall in love. Head over heels. It shocks us, comes unexpected, we seek it. Just as quickly, we fall out of love. Love hurts. Nothing is ever ours to keep. Yet I hoarded it, hoarded the memories. A reminder, a warning. Whoever comes out of love a survivor?

Beginning. Middle. End. I was bombarded by memory and the present colliding to become indistinguishable. Millions of little big bangs creating millions of beginnings. All just a series of cause and effect. The pendulum between each of the men had swung from love to pain to love to abuse to love to trauma. I sighed as I placed the relics back in the boxes, sealing them away for another time.

I'm a collector, a hoarder of memories. Take the needle and stitch. Thread together the memories. Memory is the place of second chances where we can relive moments and people from long ago that are no longer part of our lives. Borrowed memories, collective memories, mined from the personal, culled from the collective. The mind is a series of rooms, a house, glass cases in a museum of times gone by. But we are still here, still living, in the present. Unlock the door, disturb the dust and enter. I stockpiled the memories, preserved them, so I could binge on them but I had never fully digested them. Now was the time to pick them apart, to understand what they meant, and how they had affected me. How they drove me to this moment, to those lips quick to love, lips quick to anger.

Life seemed to have been a process of breaking and rebuilding. Other people had, society had, continually divided me. I was made to feel so broken that I felt irreparable. What happens when parts no longer make a whole, when they've been split unevenly? What had happened to me in the past that conditioned me to accept treatment like that? When had the language of love been so beaten out of me that I believed love and abuse belonged to the same root?

I've always been amazed at the body's ability to heal. One side of a cut that will slowly reach out to the side that has been torn away and somehow create a new whole. The way a bruise can creep, bloom into purples and coral, then disappear as if it were never really there. How a burn can make the skin crisp, melt, then dry, like a pool of lava until only a ghost mark remains of what used to be there. What scared me is how we heal on the inside. We cut things out, forget, store away pain and trauma in vaults that remain sealed for years until someone else who has the key lets it out. We never know whether it has truly healed or not.

Where did it all begin? That's what I wanted to know. Looking at the museum of my life in that room, I needed to understand the trauma in my past and why it had happened. We cultivate our own mythologies. Weaving together our own memories, memories from other people, shared ones, to create the tapestry of our own histories. Was it running through the forest barefoot? Every time I was belittled? The times I was cheated on? The words from the altar telling me I was wrong? No one knows when everything began, we are a chain of endings without knowing our exact origins. I was going to try my best to find out.

I tried to find my way back into myself again, to run my fingers along those faint internal scars to figure out who or what had caused them, and why. What is made cannot be unmade, but I could begin to understand the scars to overcome them. I propped myself up against the headboard and flipped open my laptop. I began to read. I began to think. I pushed myself into the past. I began to write.

There are many beginnings; it all depends on at what point we start to define ourselves.

Chapter Two

The park of my childhood was always divided in two, like one giant game of Bulldog. The girls were at one end, some doing handstands against the garages, others weaving daisies into crowns and sitting coroneted while making nests from freshly cut grass. With matching crimped hair and pedal pushers, they sang the latest pop songs, each one assigned their place in the band according to their looks or personality. I always thought I would be Sporty because I could do backflips like her. I wasn't asked to join.

The teenagers on the other side played football with their still-breaking voices calling to each other to pass the ball, topless torsos pearled with sweat. I watched, fascinated, as muscle shifted under skin. I had an urge to be amongst them, to know them, to touch them. I wasn't asked to join.

After the game they sat on the climbing frame, passing a cigarette. They were a gang of grazed knees and grass-stained tracksuits, the lingering smell of Lynx mixing with smoke. They sat flicking ash from their cigarettes until the streetlights came on. They held them like lollipops as if they weren't quite ready to graduate from childhood. The cherry glowed in front of mouths barely grazed with stubble. I picked a dandelion, breathed deeply and blew the wish-laden seeds onto the night's breeze to plant them somewhere else, somewhere in the future. The park turned the social division that we had been taught was right and normal into a stretch of real space.

It was the hub of the estate where each gang of friends, or family gang as mine was, played until dark. It was the place where our imaginations played out, where boys chased girls to kiss them, where we read the local gossip scrawled in pen under the slide, where arguments were settled with fights.

Bulldog was one of the ways conflicts were resolved. It was prearranged: whoever was the bulldog would know whom they had to 'catch' easily. A coalition was then formed to gang up on the ones who had insulted us. The visible prickling, the chests puffed, muscles and sinews taut and ready to pounce. The thud of bodies being slammed on the grass, the sharp gasp as air was forced from their lungs, the cry as a sly punch was given. The cheering, the shrieking, the snarling. The shift of eyes and shimmer of fear when they realised it was a set-up. Once it was over, we'd skulk off, licking wounds or peacocking with pride and retribution.

From the green sprawled the alleys and roads where we lived, all named after trees and birds. Even now, I can still remember each one, where they branched, and who lived where: ally and foe. It was a root system that we learned to navigate when running away from the man who chased us with an axe after playing Knock Door Run, where we would need to fly to if there was a fight, or the quickest route home before the streetlights came on.

Down those alleys lurked old women who twitched back their net curtains and watched us play. They whispered and wove what we did into their moth-eaten gossip-catchers, and stored them there like embroidered prey until they next saw my nan at bingo. This game was their event of the week, held every Tuesday at the hall. My nan, the queen bee, sat in the middle as the other women hovered around her. She'd laugh with a cup of tea in her hand as they told her what trouble we'd been stirring up.

Trouble was our gift as we didn't have much else. We made do with what we had to the limits of our imaginations. We invented a *dramatis personae* for the characters on the estate, for that's what they were. They weren't of reality. 'Gummy', who chased us in her slippers, gums moist and shining as she screamed at us; the man who buried children under his back gate; the man who never entered or left the bungalow with the white door and thorn bushes spilling over his garden walls.

We played It across the park where our trainers stuck in the rubbery surface like fingers in warm cookie dough, chasing growing shadows and screams until dark. We used a car bonnet to create a roof for our base, fashioning a rounders bat out of a shoe. We hunted vampires and cast spells around alley corners. We built rafts, lashing together logs and branches, and tried to sail down the river where the smallest of us was selected as tribute to test whether they'd sink or float. They always sank. During the winter we slid on tea trays down the icy hill with our scarves caught in the air and in snow flurries, my brother skidding down on his bike and breaking his arm at the bottom.

We found pennies on the street, ran to the shop to buy Black Jacks and sucked them quickly, poking out our jet-stained tongues. A few weeks later, we were barred from the same shop for calling Bab, the owner, 'Kebab'. It was a badge of pride when someone was barred from the shop; the ultimate glory was being banned for life. 'Life' – a few weeks – at that time was endless, like the woods where we ran from dawn to dusk.

The main entrance was a cemetery to the estate's junk – a precious place to us that could be plundered for everything: the rusted bike wheels crusted like halves of an orange left uneaten for too long, ripped sofas that could be dragged through the thicket and used as a throne in our base. It was the place where we tied string to tree trunks and bent branches to navigate our way through and back safely until we learned the routes as well as the streets we grew up on. We climbed trees and felt dew-tipped moss under our hands to try see where the treescape finished. It was where the teenagers allegedly had sex in a burned-out car. It was filled with drops of white during spring, then crushed blues and purples when bluebells pushed up between ferns and pines. The shadowed creeks and streams that shone pink, purple, red, like oil on water during sunsets. Mist dripped and draped on branches; light spun like sugar on leafy paths. We turned up home at night covered in mud. I never did find the other side of the woods.

However, there was always enough to keep us busy within the estate. Under the froth of apple blossom, the froth of blood from a split lip. The crunch of dried-out branches mixed with the snap of bone. There were bleeding noses, chipped teeth and brawls that happened down alleys or on the green. Doubled over, my mouth wide open, there was no noise and no air after I'd been winded from a kick to the stomach. The fist that smashed into my face. I didn't feel it until I was on the floor, staring at the scuffed trainers around me. The howling and laughing, too sinister for children. The creak of the metal chains on the park swings as they went back and forth, back and forth, back and forth as I lay alone on the green with my eye beginning to mottle in red and green and purple. The bruise crawled across my cheek like lichen. Arguments behind netted windows. The glint of broken things on the park as the sun set. The flash of a knife as I saw a man being stabbed. The glimmer of blood down the alley that he'd never use as a trail back home.

Difference forged us an identity, made us fiercely defensive and proud of where we came from and who we were, despite some of the trouble that went on. If kids from another estate came looking for trouble, we'd drive them away. The rich kids at our primary school knew not to mess with us twice after calling us skanks. When the police were called because a bin was set on fire, or because of a fight or smashed window, there would be a warning echo of 'Police!' that cascaded down the alleys to warn everyone to play a very real game of hide and seek. No matter the divisions and bullying and anger that threaded its way through the estate, there was an undying loyalty to it and a desire to protect ourselves from the hate we felt from people beyond its borders.

We guarded what was precious to us: the smell of pine and bluebells and morning, and the stickiness of resin on palms. Thorn-pricked fingers, blackberry-stained lips and jam jar fishing. On Bonfire Nights we'd all huddle together, white breath smoking from mouths, eating barbecue food, licking toffee apple remains from our lips. We ran across the frost-tipped grass screaming, shadows flickering around us, as the night exploded in colours, stars and gasps. There was a network of families where parents knew parents, grandparents knew grandparents. They would take us in even if we were locked out or offer a cup of tea despite longstanding feuds. Each street held a place of safety if we needed it. We defended our estate, and ourselves, fiercely.

The estate was a parallel world that gave me a childhood that no one else I have met outside understands. My parents gave us everything we needed; the estate gave us everything we needed. We didn't miss anything. We had open fields where the farmer chased us with a gun, my cousins to hang out with, an orchard where we were pushed over the fence to scrump apples and launch them over the fence for my grandad to catch. This is what we knew, and this is what was normal. We didn't want anything different. We didn't crave more and didn't know what we didn't have.

Normal was something we all understood. They, we, had learned all about difference at school although it wasn't on the syllabus. We were the council estate skanks. The ones who rocked up to school on the chuntering bus with the seats that always seemed to smell of smoke, shouting and swearing as we jumped off. There was giggling so hard we wet ourselves, love notes passed across classrooms, the choir, the nickname we gave to a teacher that remained long after we left. There were chairs and tables thrown, teachers bitten and escape jobs. Every time a kid from the estate leaped over the school gate there was a huge cheer as they fled down the road with the headmaster running behind them. A friend and I snuck out spoons from lunch and tried to dig a tunnel from the field under the fence to the road on the other side. We only managed a few inches. We constantly tried to escape to freedom without ever knowing what our end game would be. End game.

Teachers and other children marked us as different: *skank, pikey, chav, townie, povvo*. There was the teacher who dug her nails into our heads and shoulders and threatened to seal our mouths shut with Sellotape. The teacher who told me, aged eight, that I would grow up to be 'nothing', despite excelling in all my subjects. Just '*another* one from the estate'. There was something wrong about someone from a council estate who wanted to learn and did well academically. It was incomprehensible that some of us didn't live up to the stereotypes, so we were all branded the same: no potential, no hopes.

Teachers aren't parents. But they are there to mould, shape, educate, inspire and encourage no matter ability or background. Yet the ones we had educated us to not believe in ourselves, they taught us that we didn't deserve better. Those types of comments and behaviour stick to a child like gum under a desk. No matter how much you scrape and paint over it, the marks still linger. I was lucky that my parents encouraged us to study and learn and try. *Be better, do better, be the best,* my parents taught us, my mum's red hair falling across her face as she leaned over to help us with our homework, the encyclopaedias sent from my grandma open on the table. They knew and taught us that education and knowledge would take us elsewhere. I would be better, do better and be the best, despite what teachers, the rich kids and life threw at me.

We didn't think we were different or where we lived was different, until we were told that we were. But, just like the world outside the estate imposed a hierarchy on us, the hierarchies within it were just as ruthless and constrictive. 'Normal' was something we all understood, but we had our own definitions and regulations of what that constituted.

In some ways, the estate was governed by a meritocracy. You were judged by your own abilities to hold your own and by earning your place in the hierarchy. Survival of the fittest. In other ways, there was a strange sense of equality, whereby the usual patriarchal rules didn't apply. The girls wore boy clothes, they beat up boys twice their size and height, played football. It was all acceptable. But then there was me. I was the exception to the rule. On the streets where gender theories played out, I was the one marked as different. I was the one who pushed it too far.

It all started with a bet. I must have been around four or five and trying to do handstands. Steph, my cousin, would grip my ankles to hold me up and keep my legs straight as my arms squirmed to keep myself balanced. Eventually, she said she'd give me £1 if I could do it by myself with straight legs. I practised against walls, in the park, around the house, in my nan's living room in front of the coal-fuelled fire, in the playground until the point where I was no longer covered with grazed skin and could do a perfect handstand (I received the £1 twenty years later).

My parents encouraged me to take up gymnastics, quickly progressing from my local club to the next big town's gymnasium. It was full of people twisting and contorting in the air, thrumming hearts and muscle, full of people like me. I was home. Within a year, my coach pulled me aside and crouched down to speak with me alone.

'Michael, how old are you?'

'Seven,' I shuffled, worried I'd done something wrong.

'I've been thinking about moving you up to the senior squad. What do you think?' I looked over at the rings where they were training. They were twice my size, had been training for years, they pulled themselves up into handstands on the rings effortlessly. I couldn't even do that properly yet. You were normally supposed to be at least 15 to join the senior squad.

'Would it just be me?' He nodded and I looked over to the ball pit room where my friends played, a rainbow of balls in the air as they screamed and jumped in. It'd no longer be a game. I said I would, not knowing that once again I'd be looking in from the outside as they played together.

It meant training five days a week compared with three. The talent I had was recognised by my trainers. I was fearless and threw myself into every contortion and twist without a second thought. The fear of myself I was forced to feel in the playground was gone. I knew this was a chance to become professional, realise my talent, finally reach the edge of the woods, and escape. As I backflipped and somersaulted endlessly without fault, pulled myself to the top of the rope tied to the top of the tree in my garden, as my down-covered arms became rope-like in turn, I recognised the talent in myself. In the car at night on the way home, my mum sang to Sonique's 'It Feels So Good', the two of us screaming alongside Kelis when 'Caught Out There' came on. I sat with chalk on my hands like crushed stars determined to change my fortunes.

Aged 8 I was seen to have the talent to be a future Olympian. Steph moved from the estate around this time. The time spent together reading, writing, playing, talking about imaginary worlds was gone. I depended on her, she protected me, and without her I was isolated in my reality. I was a changeling. I wasn't like the other kids; a queer.

Poof. Faggot. Queer. Batty. Billy Elliot. Gay. Gender bender.

The talent I had was a step too far on the estate: it was the ultimate form of femininity. The parameters of gender, and sexuality, had been set from an early age. I was supposed to play with boys, but not in *that* way. I was supposed to like girls, but only in *that* way. How a boy should be was clear: football, spitting, messing around in school. There was no space for fluidity, no comprehension of digression. I didn't meet those expectations and I was told so, made to feel so, with no regrets on their part. Gymnastics marked me as the ultimate sign of deviance on the streets glittering with glass and beer cans.

It didn't matter that I dressed just like the other kids: blue, black or red tracksuit bottoms and t-shirt; I'd learned years before that some colours were dangerous. My leotard was safely hidden in my room, never to be seen by them. Or that the scuff marks on my trainers from backflips were no different to theirs from football tackles. My calloused palms were no different to theirs except mine were covered in chalk rather than oil, grease or dirt. My body looked no different to theirs, either. If anything, my musculature, strength and power were greater than those who bullied me, from the hundreds of pull-ups I did in the gymnasium to lifting my body from a seated position up through my arms into a handstand. It's strange how prejudice works: gymnastics requires almost an excess of what is typically coded masculine. The problem was that their type of masculinity was qualified and justified with the prequisite of being heterosexual: somehow, they could see something in me that I couldn't.

As clearly as I remember foraging for mushrooms in fields with my nan, card games over numerous cups of tea filled with tiny whirlpools and portents, and the buddleia covered in butterflies outside the kitchen window, I remember the names I was branded with as early as five. They called it on the streets. They called it in the playground. They called it down the woods. It echoed across the estate and in my dreams. I asked what 'gay' meant, I had no idea what it was. I was told it meant happy, but I knew from the way it was said it was nothing like that.

In that building that smelled of chalk and sweat I found refuge. For nine hours a week my body belonged to me. My body didn't mean anything beyond the boundaries I pushed it to. During those hours, I owned who I was. It was where no one knew about the estate and where I came from. In those four walls, I wasn't different; I was the same as everyone else. Beyond the estate, gymnastics wasn't queer or feminine, it was normal. If anything, it was respected for the power and strength needed to do it. I was judged on my ability and not for who or what I was. We were all equal.

I trained with military dedication: sitting in front of the TV eating my dinner doing the splits, walking around the living room on my hands and backflipping in the garden. I trained to forget and escape. The beat of my body thumping on the sprung floor became my heartbeat. If I had continued to progress at the same rate, it would have been my life. However, there was my life outside the gym that wouldn't go away or let me forget. There were two colliding forces, and only one could survive and only one could exist. It was whichever was stronger.

There was a different coach who trained the senior squad. I had met him before: a few times he'd instructed the juniors and he wrung out our young bodies like old cloth. I dreaded having him for five days a week. One of his favourite games was to make me somersault five times within a five-metre stretch of floor to perfect my execution and precision. I'd pound the floor, tuck myself in, and land with my toe inches from the edge. *Again.* I'd walk back to the start with my head still spinning. *Again.* We'd repeat and repeat until we failed or couldn't walk. His techniques made some of the other kids cry. I refused to cry. I was taught not to.

The bullying outside was equally relentless. 'Where's your tutu, poof?' They mock-pirouetted, pranced and leaped across the green with limp hands, telling me to plié – how it must have been easy as I didn't have a dick – their laughter wrapping me up like ribbons on a pointe shoe. In the classroom at school, on the bus on the way back home, scrawled in red across the wood under the slide. I tried to be like them: I no longer did routines on the green; I attempted to play football. The bigger they are, the harder they'll fall, I was told. I made them fall and they made me fall twice as hard. I would be just like them. It didn't work. I carried that mark throughout the rest of my childhood. They didn't forget and wouldn't let me.

Something inside was eating me, sucking the light and energy into some epic darkness that I didn't know how to escape from. It was something even I couldn't tightrope or vault over like I'd been trained. I stood on the mat edge staring at breeze block walls without energy, without purpose, without the wired twitching I used to have before taking my turn. I still executed every routine perfectly, but it was like I'd been programmed, it had become mechanical. I ran through the motions instead of into freedom. My shadow leapt across the building as I somersaulted and flung myself from the high bar, and that shadow crept home with me and cradled my heart. They made it so gymnastics was no longer home. So, I quit. They had won.

I still remember the day, 26 June 1999. It was a few weeks before my ninth birthday and a few months before I was due to have my first competition. I had been relentlessly learning the routine. I ensured that every landing pivoted seamlessly to the next move, every toe was pointed, every launch was powerful, my back always curved, everything was perfected even down to how I presented myself to the judges before beginning the routine. To this day, I still stand in the same way.

I didn't realise at the time how much gymnastics provided me an escape from the bullying, from the loneliness I felt. It gave me the space to escape their brands even just for a few hours. When I performed on the floor, vaulted metres into the air, my body dissolved. On the high bar, the metal cold under my chalk-dusted leathered palms, the callouses permanently grafted to my hands. The thrum of the bar as I rotated and rotated around it, my legs and toes pointed, an arrow through the air gathering speed and momentum. The rush of air, my head clear, my eyes focused. Pulling up to a pike and balancing at the top of the bar in a handstand, swinging round one more time, my hands slid from the bar and I launched into the air and for the briefest of moments I was a central point of light. I detached from my body. I wasn't the queer, the poof who played with girls, the local Billy Elliot. Without gymnastics, there were times I wanted to commit suicide.

It was driven by an overwhelming sense of exhaustion. I was exhausted from trying. From being me. It demanded so much energy and concentration to be someone else, to make sure they didn't see how it affected me. Ultimately, it did. I knew why they bullied me – they made it as clear as could be. I just didn't understand or know why being different was wrong. I logged and stored all of it away in a vault and carried on like we had been taught. I knew how much I was loved by my family, but it was the world that made me feel utterly alone.

If I should die before I wake, I pray the Lord my soul to take. I prayed it most nights. Hoping He would take me, asking Him why He had made me like this, asking Him to make me normal (little did I know I was trying to pray the gay away). As I curled up in bed, I prayed and prayed to be cleansed of whatever this difference was. I asked myself those same questions that the other kids asked me.

I wanted to know why I was different. Girls like boys, so should I have been one? I wondered if I'd been transplanted into a boy's body, if I'd been born in the wrong body, if something had gone wrong with me in the womb. What had made me this way? Why I was so different? I had no answers, just the knowledge that whatever it was that made me this way, it was bad. With the duvet pulled over my head I thought how I didn't belong.

I quit gymnastics because I thought it would make the bullying stop. The other kids made the decision for me and took the choice away. I learned a year later that the coach had left. Part of me when I learned that thought maybe I could go back; it wasn't too late. But it wouldn't have stopped the other kids as their brand was permanent, like the gossip written on the wood under the slide. Even years after I quit, they still called me Billy Elliot. I'd tell them that I didn't even do it anymore and that he did ballet, not gymnastics. It didn't make a difference.

I was taught to recite that age-old phrase, *Sticks and stones may break my bones, but words can never hurt me.* Words can hurt; they have the ability to shape and destroy. They rooted a deep sense of shame in who I am. They conditioned me to believe I wasn't normal, that difference was inherently wrong. After Steph left the estate, I didn't know anyone else like me, who had similar interests. I didn't see my reality reflected in books or film. It reinforced that being gay was wrong. I was told I was gay. I was told that was wrong.

I knew I felt something, I didn't understand it or know what it was. I knew I was different to them, but naming, vocalising or shaping that difference into something concrete – a word, a gesture, an action – wasn't possible. They were all so wise; they could put a name to it. Police it, force it, control it. I didn't think there was anything different about me until they told me so. Difference is born on the lips.

To be accepted as a man and convince others of our manhood,[1] beyond physiology, we have to perform the gender codes[2] we're taught as children through our physicality, interests, clothes and behaviour. I didn't fit on either side of the green: I read books, I was a gymnast, I had ripped-out magazine pages of Britney Spears on my walls. My acts didn't convince the other children of my 'membership' to their type of masculinity. The smallest acts became the biggest gender subversion. I was branded as feminine and, by proxy, gay. Gender slipped into sexuality.

Through the relentless bullying I experienced throughout my childhood, the policing of my identity, I was forced to adopt a new skin, a new identity that aligned with what was accepted and 'normal'. I no longer played with dolls, I no longer wore pink or colours associated with girls. It didn't make a difference. On the outside I was no different, they figured something inside wasn't right. Delicacy and sensitivity clung to me like some perfumed mist despite the coils of muscle it stuck to. Its sweet scent made people alert, to look twice at me, made them want to hurt the softness in me. As a child growing up on an estate, I became that *other* so the other children felt less fragile and more empowered in a world where we were already considered less. The unhappiness and ugliness they felt: they wanted me to feel it more.

I understand now how the homophobic slurs the kids on the estate called me were a way for them to signify their own heterosexuality and dominance. The feminine was regarded as the antithesis of masculine, weak and emotional, which made me a lesser man, gay. It allowed them to police what they didn't view as acceptable male acts. Mine broke the boundaries they set and knew. My gender expression was viewed as both feminine and homosexual, and they policed this identity to validate and reassure their own. The gender signifiers that are enforced on us from birth are powerful.

They give us rules, codes, an understanding of how we organise ourselves and how to behave. I broke them so they broke me.

The ones who identified my sexuality before I understood what sexuality was, the people who expected me to behave a certain way because of where I grew up, helped themselves to my identity. It belonged to them. They policed me out of my skin and made me a refugee from my body. I was queer. Not that this was something I understood or recognised in myself. But those girls braiding their hair, the boys swapping Marlboros seemed to know.

The public image of the working class so often depicts violence, big families, delinquency; it is full of negative representations of lazy, 'benefit-sponging' people. We're considered inarticulate, unintelligent. Yet, I always remember every single person working; I remember happy families and happily married parents. The true community is never shown. How we protect each other and our space, our stories. Even as an adult coming back to the estate, I might bump into someone who knew me when I was young, recognise that I'm from my family and tell me stories about my mum, aunts and uncles of when they were young, or ask about my nan. We are full of complexities and contradictions, but we are full of fire, full of stories. Stories that deserve to be told. The world, the media, people need to alter how working-class people are depicted and treated. We're taught to be small, that we're no good, that we should aspire to be nothing. Even though the kids in that community caused me pain, there were other systems society put in place that bonded us together.

The estate taught me to be tenacious and resilient. To fight for myself, to defend myself. It taught me the value of family and friends, and to fight for them. It taught me to work hard for everything because nothing was ever going to be given to me. It taught me to fight for opportunities, to take them, be grateful for them. It taught me to take a punch, figuratively and literally, and how to get back up. Life was and is full of punches, and I don't know how I would have survived if I'd grown up elsewhere. The estate taught me not to give up, not to cry when things get difficult, but to figure a way through it. Childhood wasn't always easy, but I wouldn't trade it for anything else.

It shaped me into who I am now; when embarking on this journey, those memories on the estate were the first to come to my mind when trying to understand what had happened in the past that got me to where I am in the present. If I look back, this is the point in my life I always go to when I think of trauma, when I was first singled out and forced to feel different. It played a pivotal and instrumental part in my life and shaped who I was and the perception I had of myself. It taught me shame, self-hate, difference. The othering we face as children, the bullying, and the invalidity we're forced to feel towards our sexuality or gender carries into our adulthood as trauma, making us feel inadequate or displaced in a heterosexual world where we've always been told we don't belong. It instils in us a sense that being gay and the feminine are wrong.

Misogynistic and queerphobic insults are by no means isolated to the working class. It wouldn't have mattered if my parents had moved us to a different place, homophobia isn't bound to estates. Difference will be found regardless of geography. Across all classes and cultures, difference is weaponised as a way to ostracise and shame people who do not conform or express their gender and sexuality to the hegemonic ideal that we're taught as children. Such differences are a way to bully people into constrictive boxes.

Living on a rural estate, there was little variety or exposure to a range of heterosexual masculinities. I didn't know anyone who was gay, let alone know of such a thing as an LGBTQ+ community. As a result, there was greater pressure to adhere to binary gender and sexuality roles, and greater vilification if you did not. I lived in a place where the countryside and the estate provided endless opportunities for us to explore, except when it came to identity. Not being validated or seen or understood, not feeling safe in who we are growing up when we are at such formative ages can be destructive and traumatic. It constantly displaces us from feeling okay in who we are, when all we are trying to do is find belonging as a child in a world that is already scary.

If we're to survive these conditions, we have to metamorphose into what is viewed as acceptable. Conformity means survival. To avoid the bullying, losing the love of family, we put on a different skin to hide the real one. From the earliest of ages, I was forced to assume a public and interior identity. I set my story against theirs: theirs won. I have had so many beginnings and so many endings as I've needed to survive with different versions of myself. I wrote stories and versions of myself to survive because the pain if I hadn't would have been more unbearable than it already was.

I was taught to be ashamed of this interior identity because of society's expectations of masculinity and sexuality. It conditioned the deepest shame, the belief that I was wrong because being gay was wrong. This type of trauma shame – the shame you are made to feel after experiencing trauma – can result in self-hatred,[3] while also causing traumatic shame – to feel traumatised by the shame you feel. Over the years, the mimicking of someone and something else, hiding one's true self, the internalised self-hatred, had done untold damage to my mental and emotional health. Bullying and othering lay the foundations for many issues that LGBTQ+ people become susceptible to later in life. This type of trauma is 'shame-based' and makes people 'have core beliefs that they are unlovable, that if people knew what they were really like they would leave'.[4] This can play a part in forming trauma bonds in abusive relationships, clinging to a love even if it is abusive or toxic and overcompensating to keep the abuser, as there is a deep-rooted sense of worthlessness.

Even now, depending on the situation and who I'm with, an infinite number of adjustments, changes and corrections occur in my body. I recalibrate my movements, my thoughts, my words, my accent; I switch roles to be the masculine working-class boy that I was supposed to be. I realign unconsciously to behave according to what's expected, to the words that were written so deeply on my body as a child. Like a tightrope walker, I perform the perfect balancing act, above a pit where light and shadow play.

I often think of the life they stole from me. Not specifically the life I could have had with gymnastics, but the escape, the thing that was mine. I often think of the life I was forced to live and how differently my confidence and self-respect would be now without their words stitched on my skin. How might pride feel without pain? How different could my relationships have been – could I have avoided the abuse I suffered in some of them?

The people around me growing up rejected and denied my identity and forced me to do the same. Validation is core to constructing who we are, as well as building a healthy connection with ourselves physically and emotionally. Yet when we are rejected and denied validation for who we are, it ostracises us from the world around us, makes us believe we don't belong there, we don't fit, we aren't normal. How do we reconcile what the world reflects, what we've been forced to reflect with the face that is unseen in the mirror? There's always been a face in the mirror that collides with my own.

Do the kids on the estate and my primary school teachers remember who I am and what they did? I doubt it. I remember their names, their words, how it made me feel, how it changed me and how it affects me today. What part of society deems it okay for a child to be terrified of the world around them, to be terrified of who they are, to feel like they don't belong? All because of structures, paradigms, stereotypes and prejudices the world has created about their gender, sexuality, class, ability or race. All based on an idealism that is no more than a veil to wield power.

Masculinity that intersects with a minority status is so often viewed as inferior. The enforced subordination to the dominant, white, heterosexual and middle-class masculinity conditioned me to see myself and my roots as worthless and shameful. There is an inherent right that comes with white, middle- and upper-class male heterosexuality that is not granted to the rest of us. Intersections of race compound so much – I know how my whiteness has lessened the sting in many ways.

There is an inherent pathway, and if we do not stay on it we are thrown to the wolves. Their structures and codes are metaphors for power. We as working class, we as queer, disrupt that story and weaken the hierarchies they have imposed. The council estate kid who succeeds, the queer that goes on to own and love their sexuality. We have our own power in subversion, in digression, in disruption, in protest. It shows our strength that time after time we rise and we transform despite the trauma, the subordination, the hate.

My childhood was marked by a strict adherence to the gender binary and a homogenous view of how masculinity should be expressed. In the past decade there has been a shift in accepting a variety of gender expressions. There is greater representation of fluidity and the gender spectrum. Gender and sex and sexuality are becoming recognised as distinguishable; one does not necessarily always follow the other.

However, this is by no means a battle won. LGBTQ+ youth are still significantly more likely to attempt or consider suicide than their heterosexual peers; one report found that 44 per cent of LGBTQ young people had thought about suicide.[5] This is not necessarily the fault of family, but the structures society puts in place where queer youth feel there is no hope for them. From our parents, peers and friends through to the media, we are confronted, pressurised and shamed into a homogeneous version of masculinity and the gender binary. Two distinct narratives where adherence and conformity are expected. It took years of self-work, reflection and dedication to understand my worth, to be proud of where I come from and who I am. It took just as long to begin to reject what I had been conditioned to believe about myself, learning that happiness doesn't equate to normal. The traces of the trauma and abuse I went through as a child for being gay and working-class remain wrapped tightly around my DNA. It didn't come without consequence. It laid the foundations for pain and hurt much worse later. It was one of the many beginnings that set this story in motion.

From my bedroom windowsill as the nights grew longer and summer was dying, I'd watch the swifts cut up the last of the light. A black 'V' in the pinks and oranges, an arrow impaling the sky, an arrow to the future. Their last dance of the year before disappearing in the lacy shadows. It was a reminder that a new season was dawning, time was turning, the future was an arrow in the dark. At some point it would be my turn to join them, past the woods and disappear beyond the horizon.

Chapter Three

It began with a kiss, as it does in a fairy tale or a movie. I almost hadn't gone: I was tired, anxious, couldn't be bothered with another failed date. My housemate and her friend encouraged me to go. It was an unexpected surprise. We spent the evening talking about films, as he was studying screenwriting, and books and life and politics. Outside Angel Tube station in the rain, as we said our goodbyes the lamplight showering us, the fizz rising up in my stomach, we kissed. That's how this story begins.

We passed mornings in bed together talking and laughing, discussing his scripts and my short stories. In my bed, away from the world, with only the sunlight to creep in and listen to our whispers and secrets. I listened with my head on his chest and my eyes closed as the sun filtered up and across the room to the point where I saw orange behind my lids. He held me tightly every time we woke, his deep laugh reverberating across the branches of my ribs and into my roots. There, pressed against him, I was finally safe in another's arms. His kisses were the most tender, always as if he were kissing me for the first or last time. Passion jumped from the lips and I let it grow, finally allowing myself to love and be loved in return.

He was due to move back to America to finish college and we lived every moment like it was the first and the last. We skimmed stones into the sea on Brighton Beach and held each other on the pebbles, buffeted by the coastal wind, as we sang our song into each other, 'When We Were Young'. With my face against his chest, he couldn't see the streaks of salt that could have been tears or sea.

Adele was right, it was just like a movie. Everything was too perfect. Every time I saw him, I was filled with warmth, the safety I felt when he held me and said my name. I allowed myself to dream, allowed myself to love, I dared to sink into the possibility of a future. I dared myself to love and to deserve love. I imagined children and marriage, the home we would make together.

Time doesn't wait for anyone. Not even love. The time had come for him to return home. We had dinner, walked through Soho, ate ice cream, kept talking, kept walking. Trying to delay the inevitable. We held each other outside the barriers in Tottenham Court Road. People racing to get places, moving, another destination to get to. We wanted everything to stop. Not wanting the minutes to pass for his flight to come. For there to be no further destination. Not wanting to be anywhere else except in the other's arms.

As I walked through the barriers and looked back at him alone, waving, I felt my heart hurt for the man, for the time we'd had together, for the relationship that we had built. For the love I was able to give, accepting the love I finally deserved. Even now, years later, when I walk through that station my body remembers the ghost of his body pressed against me, his arms around me, his smile as he crossed the road to greet me. He ascended to the street and I descended to the earth, not knowing where we would come out and meet again.

We agreed to keep going long distance, not wanting to end what we had. He came to visit in the summer for a few weeks. We slotted back together like no time had passed. Yet, weeks later, we clung to each other on a platform. One train went by. And another. Another. I twisted my fingers into the grey jumper he loved that I said he could keep. We tried to laugh and smile between tears and sniffs as we'd be seeing each other again, soon, sometime in the future. The doors slid open and shut. Make a choice, jump on, hop off. Mind the closing doors. Mind the closing doors. Each one an opportunity snapping shut. The clock was ticking, time was running out. Trying to stop it, stall it, we were mining for time.

'Let me see those baby blues. One more time.' He held my head between his hands and smiled, and I tried to smile back. The smile where you can feel your lips curl and wobble from trying not to cry. When you hold your breath in your chest so as not to cry out. He kissed me. Like it was the first time, like it was the last time. Like he always did.

I'd been miserable in the job I had taken to pay the bills after I'd been made redundant from my first job in publishing. Every morning I woke up with stomach pains that felt like I was being stabbed repeatedly so I couldn't move; I'd hunch over at the bus stop, leaning against the wall to hold myself up. A best friend from university, a performance artist, and her partner, had uprooted from London earlier that year to find a new life in Avignon, creating a home, studio and performance space in one. I'd tried and tried to find another job in publishing with no luck. When they asked me to be their beta artist-in-residence I uprooted and followed them. I needed to figure out what I wanted to do with my life, what made me happy, to actually stop and rest.

In the city where popes had once pottered around, with an unfinished bridge that had no ending, I wrote and wrote and wrote. I didn't care what came out, I just needed to do the thing I loved. As part of the residency, I had to give a performance of something I had written at an art night they were holding with the theme 'Post-Mortem'. One of the short stories I wrote was set in a bath. A tale of love and loss and memory and time. Lost love and lost time. So, I gave a reading in Speedos in a claw-foot tub.

I breathed out and unfolded a beginning, an ending; my post-mortem. Looking back, there was something prescient about that night. Examining the carcass of my previous life, plunging into the waters and coming out as someone else, baptised into something new. *There are many beginnings; it all depends on at what point we start to define ourselves,* I read. From water we are born, in water we are reborn.

On the last day before I returned to the UK, we drove through the countryside in their Mustang listening to Serge Gainsbourg, sunglasses on to help our hangovers. We stopped in Lacoste full of archways and mossed alleys that disappeared, where the clock tower's hands didn't move. We stood outside the Marquis de Sade's castle, bolted shut, his secrets and fantasies chained up once again. My friend kissed a sculpture, the Marquis's head in a cage, and left her lips imprinted, joining the hundreds of other dead kisses. I looked out to the countryside, the sharp blue of the sky, the twisted vineyards like planted spines, and the whole place was silent. The clock tower didn't ring out, there was no wind and no sound. The whole world was frozen. There next to Sade's chamber where bodies and words fell to his whim, I knew what I had to do. I could no longer flee the past.

I knew I had to work with books again. I sent out hundreds of applications and didn't get an interview for any. On that last try, months later, I got a job for a charity called First Story. They send professional writers into schools that serve low-income communities to run creative writing workshops with students. At the end of the year a collection of each school's work is published. Not only does it serve to increase communication and literacy skills, but also to give young people from diverse, working-class backgrounds the confidence that their stories and voices are powerful and important.

In the four months I worked for them, I read stories of travel, love, loss, friendship. I tasted food from all corners of the earth, languages and dialects swelled at the root of tongues and on the page. From the hundreds of stories, memoirs and poetry I read, the lasting memory was the sense of pride and celebration for who they were and where they came from. There were LGBTQ+ young people, young people who protested against social and political injustice, writers with one parent, no parents, who had escaped war or lived on a council estate. These were works that glorified the diversity of their origins and selves. The way our backgrounds should be glorified.

The writers going out to the schools helped instil pride and worth and passion in thousands of children, and taught them the power and importance of their difference. I was taught shame for it. I thought how different my confidence and self-esteem could have been if my teachers had taught me to love myself and my background instead of telling me I'd be no one purely because I came from a council estate. How this could make the difference to so many others who were told they were different. I cried at my desk at the love each of these children had for themselves and their world.

There was a legion of young writers who had the confidence to share their narratives and roots, narratives and origins that do not align with the ones that dominate the bookshelves.

It felt like I had come full circle. As a boy I craved stories that reflected my world and experiences, which showed the strange, chaotic and wonderful people and places I developed alongside and inhabited. Now, as an adult, I was publishing work by a new generation of young, working-class people who were sharing their stories, without shame or fear or prejudice, for the world to experience. I didn't have those stories growing up, which has been a driving force for my own writing. The good, the bad, the ugly, the beautiful moments and people that come from both of my identities. Writing about them has allowed me to process what has happened to me, to understand them better, to help others understand them better. It's what has driven me to write this book.

For me, the most important point for any working-class or queer person, regardless of being a writer or not, is that we must celebrate our difference, be proud of where we have come from and what it has instilled in us. At that desk, I was forced to reckon with the book, media and art forms, and how special it was to see stories similar to my own reflected back. It's vital for our self-worth to see that we have a place in the world. We need to write our own stories, not the ones given to us. It's vital for others to understand us, to break down prejudices and fears. It made me question and reflect on what was missing. What had these art forms, which had given me hope and new worlds, taken away from my sense of self?

Books, without a doubt, have saved me many times throughout my life. Growing up, I imagined stories in my mind as outside I couldn't live them. Books made up the pole that kept me balanced and stopped me falling into the pit I had to tightrope over daily. The pit in my mind, the pit the world had created under me. They gave me new worlds, people, ideas and spaces beyond the one I had. Places and people to aspire to be like, worlds I dreamed I would live in beyond the parameters of the council estate and the paradigms and rules it was governed by. I'd fill out my library allowance to the maximum, birthday and Christmas lists would be dominated by the books I wanted. My cousin and I would go between

Waterstones and WHSmith, touching spines and book covers and spending our pocket money.

Literature gives us many things: hope, escapism, relief. Most of all, it provides understanding. It humanises us, shares our vulnerabilities, gives a different vision. It demonstrates our complexities and encourages us to confront the realities of different lives. Books gave me the courage and the inspiration that I could change my life and showed me there was another world beyond the one I had been given.

What books didn't provide, however, was a reflection of my day-to-day reality growing up. I had no examples that showed me that who I was or where I came from was interesting enough to write stories about or was simply normal. In the hundreds of books I read as a child, none of the characters came from a council estate. There were none who were working-class and gay. Books, which had given me refuge in so many ways, failed to show me, and countless others, that we weren't alone or strange. Alone on the council estate with no one else like me, I scoured book after book to find validation and comfort that I wasn't the only one out there. I struggled to find, or was too scared to ask for, books that combined working-class and gay voices, people who did not conform to norms. These books were not accessible or something I could ask for without revealing my sexuality growing up. But even now, as an adult, without the fear or shame I had when I was young, there is still not enough to positively show working-class queerness in all its forms.

I was introduced to *Oranges Are Not the Only Fruit* by Jeanette Winterson when I was seventeen by the guy who would become my first boyfriend. I ordered it online like it was something illegal. When it arrived, I rushed to my room to unpack it and hid it in my room so there wasn't the chance of someone else finding it. It became my bible. It didn't matter that the protagonist was a woman; the point was that I saw a reflection of myself in someone else. The streets she lurked on, the overbearing and continuous guilt of religion condemning her to damnation for loving another person. Her love of books and writing that she had to keep secret. A life that aligned with my own. Often, on my bed, I would be curled up, questioning whether I was normal, until that book allowed me to slowly unfurl. That book gave flesh to the shadows in the gaps of my imagination; it realised the people out in the world that had been faceless and storyless. Through reading, I revealed the truth about other people in the world; through reading, I revealed the truth to myself.

However, this book seemed to be the exception rather than the rule. Over thirty-five years since its publication, it's still not common to find a protagonist that is gay and working class. In art made by middle- and upper-class people where working-class characters do appear, they are used as titillation. A way to access a dangerous underworld that is so far-flung from the safe middle/upper-class world. Or even a personal project to help save, redeem or better the working-class man. We're forever grateful for the middle-class saviour. We're not celebrated for who we are, but mere tools to drive the wealthier man's decadence, guilt or sexual desires via people viewed as other. The working-class gay man is denied the right to be explored or fulfilled. Or he simply ends up dead.

On my way back from Avignon, I cried reading *Giovanni's Room*. Perhaps it affected me so greatly because it reflected so much of my own life. The intensity and emotion between Giovanni and David reflected my first relationship; like David, I escaped to another country to be so far removed from the suppressive heteronormative environment of my adolescence in order to finally feel free and safe to live my true self. It's a searing and devastating examination of same-sex desire, love and humanity. It encapsulates what so many queer people go through in feeling, and being, alienated in the environment and culture they're a product of. It highlights the way in which so many of us have had to, or continue to have to, navigate between the public and the private in order to pass as heterosexual out of shame or necessity, and the struggle we endure to find safe places to live out our true selves.

David represents so many of our experiences in feeling forced to perform an inherited masculinity, which is intrinsically tied to heterosexuality. It allows him to 'pass' in public as heterosexual, a mimicry I have also felt compelled to perform. Our own identities are shaped by the culture and society we inhabit. We are a product of that, which makes us feel alienated from our own bodies and identities that we are, or were, forced to embody in comparison with who we are inside. It creates a constant tension between who we are and who we should be. This tension inhibits, restricts and binds, and can lead to the formation of internalised homophobia because who we really are is the antithesis of what we were brought up to be. Our true selves, homosexuality, is the corruption of the image we were shown, the image we were given, the image of what we were expected to be.

David can return to his white, hetero, middle-class experience and life. He has the possibility and luxury to decide whether to live a life of normalcy and safety over happiness. He has been brought up with a certain expectation and model of masculinity, one which homosexuality opposes. Homosexuality makes him fragile, emotional, weak, feminine, less of a man. David ultimately chooses to return to his former life, one that reflects his original value set. Working-class Giovanni is given no such grace to escape where he comes from, the world that he lives in. He has no wealth, no accepting family; he cannot, and refuses to, pass as something he is not. At the end he is executed. He cannot survive in the world and nor can their love survive these internal and external pressures.

Reading more queer literature, I started to understand that there is a shared thread used repeatedly to the detriment of the working-class community. Working-class gay characters are cast aside for lovers and friends who match the rich protagonist's income bracket, values and standing. They can return to the cultured world they previously inhabited and assimilate back into safety as a more 'developed' and worldly person after their exploits, while the working-class gay man remains in their world, used and abandoned. The working-class queer character is nothing more than a prop for the narrator's desire for fun in the demi-monde, never fully formed, given a voice or seen as a real person, merely a vehicle for physical gratification, defined by physicality and masculinity. Such tropes reduce gay, working-class men to nothing more than murderers, drug-sellers, or aggressive, voiceless caricatures who have no agency, no validity or worth. They are fetishised, transgressive, dangerous, hypersexual or simply end up dead. They adhere to a hegemonic masculinity that the narrator longs for in themselves to overcome internalised homophobia. They're used to validate their own masculinity or confront the internal struggles from their childhoods and fathers. None of the relationships last, they're doomed because of self-hate, shame and society.

I saw their effect in myself: the times I would shut down a relationship before it started because I didn't feel like I was good enough for them, that they would judge me for where I came from; I couldn't understand why they were with me, how we would navigate being together – just never believed that the relationship could last.

These were books that were lauded and deemed revolutionary for their time. Yes, they reflected the realities of the gay world, of the working class, but only the negative. With each word, with each character, I saw the same words that were used to describe me as a kid on the estate: degenerate, dangerous, ambitionless. There was no complexity to these characters, no sense of the community that I had experienced or the intricacies of what being working class means. I saw the gay men whose worth was as a quick fuck, not entitled to love, respect or happiness. These books show a small minority of wealthy gay men that are too often served as protagonists or pin-ups in culture and far removed from the reality of everyday gay men.

Some of these authors lived through periods in which homosexuality was illegal and heavily discriminated against. They were showing the realities of the gay world. Their books did show the aggression and violence that I saw on the streets of my childhood. However, they didn't show the love, the intricacies and the community of both working-class and gay people. How both communities are suppressed in different ways but stick together, fight for each other, fight for liberty and opportunity. I have seen both communities fight and protest and march for better lives; people who have had to do so share a unique space for love and compassion that is so often forgotten.

More recently writers like Ocean Vuong, Paul Mendez and Jon Ransom have written books with working-class gay protagonists. They're searing, incredible insights into immigration, sex work, religion and learning to love who you are. In them, I saw people and events and smells and sounds and feelings that were similar to my own. Mohsin Zaidi's memoir, *A Dutiful*

Boy, is about growing up as a gay Muslim man in a working-class family. His journey is that of a British Asian man, which makes it different to mine, and yet many of his experiences align so much to my own story. He examines the intersections of class, sexuality and religion, while also showing the beauty and complexity found there and how working-class people do go on to achieve more than society expects. We need more representation like this.

Carlos Cortes argues that 'the news and the entertainment media "teach" the public about minorities, other ethnic groups and societal groups, such as women, gays, and the elderly'.[1] When the overwhelming portrayal is negative, what does that do to us internally in terms of how we view ourselves and our relationships? How does it impact the rest of society's views of our communities?

While our community still faces injustice and discrimination, do we as gay people not need to see stories of the love and hope that we deserve? Do we as working-class people not deserve stories where we can succeed without a middle-class saviour? People who aren't like us miss out on experiencing what class and sexuality mean in different contexts. It feels like trauma and abuse and nihilism and pain is confined to the working class, to us beyond the heteronormative. Is the middle class explored and depicted in the same way? Can we not find any beauty whatsoever in the working class? Our art forms say something different. Society, and literature, still overwhelmingly perpetuate these paradigms and perceptions. We are denied a space at the table to tell a different story, to celebrate our true stories and challenge those views. The working-class person beyond the white and heteronormative even more so.

It is important to show verisimilitude of what it means to be gay and/or working class. We also need to show the beauty of those communities, not just trauma and pain. We have moved from a vacuum of little or no representation to one that perpetuates stereotypes or reinforces the negativity we feel about ourselves or others force us to feel. We need to consider our legacy and what we leave behind, what we choose to reflect about working-class and gay people. We need representation but we also need positive representation. We have a responsibility to leave a canon where we find the beauty and pride in where we come from, who we are, what we can aspire to and what we deserve, a love and a life we all should have. Not what society believes and tells us we deserve.

Cortes further argues that representation has 'a particularly powerful educational impact on people who have little or no direct contact with members of the groups being treated'.[2] I grew up with no exposure to or knowledge of gay culture or people. What I consumed as I grew and began to explore what it meant to be gay through art and media had a profound effect on who I was, on my self-esteem. They perpetuated the story I had imposed on me by peers, teachers, colleagues my entire life: that working-class people are nothing more than street rats who don't deserve the opportunity to progress or better themselves. The doomed love stories that I had experienced – I had lived them and they were reinforced in books, and the more I exposed myself to this idea, the more I believed that this was what I deserved. This was the narrative given to me as a gay man. When my self-esteem had already been damaged by the world around me, these types of books continued to do the same thing to my self-perception.

We didn't know then that it was going to end, but there was only one ending for us in the movies, in fairy tales. All of these endings are predestined, pre-written, inexorable. They're written in books and played out on screens, and I lived them out in real life. Just like the movies. We were creating a time capsule; we were racing towards an expiry date. There's always an expiry date for love. It wouldn't be a story without the one that got away. It ended with a kiss, like it always does in a fairy tale or a movie. It woke me up to the realities of my world.

If I had known that standing together on that platform would be the last time I saw him, I would have held on longer, breathed in his smell deeper, held his face and taken a photograph that wouldn't fade, said something stupid to make him laugh one more time so I could feel the deepness of it in my bones. As the Tube disappeared towards Heathrow, I was left alone on the platform with my arms wrapped around myself even though it was summer. As he was taken further away from me, back to America, I knew deep down that we wouldn't see each other again. I knew we couldn't keep doing long distance. It was a love that couldn't surmount borders and country lines and oceans. It couldn't be sustained over bandwidths and pixels. I'd written that story before.

'Let me see those baby blues. One more time,' he asked just before the cam froze and the call dropped. I'd broken off the relationship. It wasn't just the distance, I felt like he was too good for me. That it would all end in ruin, so I would ruin it before that happened. I didn't deserve his love, so I rejected it. The trauma shame experienced in childhood bloomed in adulthood, making me feel unlovable, so I self-destructed. I thought I had broken the cycle with him. A love that was healthy and strong and reciprocated. We become what we are told. I dared myself to love, and I lost the game. He didn't know that my eyes are grey when I'm sad because he'd never made me sad. It seemed to be my thing: love lost and found over a cam.

Months later, with summer's heat and love long gone, I ran up the steps to the Curzon in Bloomsbury in the rain to meet friends to watch a film. We watched *Call Me by Your Name*, one of the few times I'd ever seen two queer leads in a mainstream film. Oliver, a graduate student, goes to Italy to study with Elio's father. Over the course of the film, there is a constant push and pull as each deny and fear their mutual attraction. Eventually, they overcome this at the last minute, finally fulfilling their desire for one another before Oliver returns to America where he ultimately marries his girlfriend. Oliver returns to the safety of perceived heterosexuality over the happiness he could have had in a gay relationship with Elio.

I cried in the dark as Italian landscapes and summer bloomed across the screen; I cried as first love bloomed and withered just as quickly as the season. I cried when I left the cinema. I cried the forty-minute bus journey from Bloomsbury back to Dalston as other passengers shuffled and tried not to stare at me. I cried for the love that would never be finally realised, the time they wasted, the memories they wouldn't make. I cried because it was a doomed relationship, one returning to his country never knowing if they'd see the other again, just like my own time in Italy. I cried for how it reflected my own first gay experience, so young and unaware under the blazing sun of an Italian summer. I cried for the first time I experienced love and how it had withered into something toxic and mean. I cried for the love I had not long lost, the love I let get away. I cried for the love that had returned to America almost a year before, never to be seen again. I cried for all the gay relationships, my own past relationships that couldn't survive. I mourned for the future loves that would suffer the same fate.

Moonlight explores masculinity and sexuality through the lives of two Black men, Kevin and Chiron. Barry Jenkins created a searing depiction of the damage masculinity can do to a man who finds himself at the intersections of race, class and sexuality, and its ability to inhibit someone living out their true self and sexuality. Chiron, who lives on an impoverished neighbourhood in Miami, is called 'faggot' for being different to the boys he grows up with. His friend, Kevin, tells him he can't let the others think he's 'soft'. It pushed me through time and space and memory to the child me backflipping across the green to the shouts of 'queer' and 'poof'. As a teenager, Chiron has a brief sexual encounter with Kevin. He is then beaten up for his sexuality, for not living up to what they expect a man to be. Years later Chiron and Kevin reunite, where Chiron reveals he hasn't had another sexual encounter with a man since that first one together on the beach. Constrained by their own inner turmoil and external stigma and pressure, which compounds the trouble the characters face, they cannot live out what is inside, their story has no beginning and no ending.

Just like my childhood, Kevin and Chiron inhabit a hostile space where their love and sexuality cannot be tolerated. There are specific masculine codes and structures they must live by in order to survive. These were policed by the other children who noticed that Chiron did not conform to their type of masculinity. Just like in my childhood, there was no room for deviance, you hide and conform to get by. Your relationships with others and yourself ultimately suffer from it. You deny yourself to cope and cope with the pain. They are not given the opportunity or luxury to escape their roots and shed the box they had been placed in. They are forever condemned to have 'What if?' linger on their lips.

Their experience as Black men in America is entirely different to my own life, but I found similarities that rang true. They feel the pressure to live up to what constitutes a 'man' in their environment. Feelings that defy the parameters of what it means to be a man in a rough housing estate. They hide who they are, they cannot live out their true selves, and their relationship can never be fulfilled. Beaten and bullied and pressurised to conform to the expectations of what it means to be a working-class male.

In these films, we see white, middle-class gay men accepted by family or returning to the safety of heterosexuality, while Black working-class men are portrayed inhabiting a hostile environment unable to escape the guilt and shame. They are destined to be trapped in their box, unable to escape the council estate, unable to live out their sexuality. It makes it look like homophobia and trauma are confined to the working-class world and other intersections. Thankfully, I did not face this same rejection when I came out to my family – working-class tropes played out on screen or in books don't always translate to real life. It took me a long time to do it because all the stories told me it would only end badly. Working-class boys deserve to see happy coming-out tales.

The media and arts are driven by conflict. It's a fundamental component to any narrative, used to keep an audience invested in the plot and characters. It helps drive development and emotion. Life isn't a clear narrative arc. There are many beginnings, middles and ends. Our days and lives are filled with multiple climaxes. A climax, in theory, is meant to be at the end of something but how does that apply to the theory of beginning, middle and end in life? Life isn't as neatly packaged as it is in the arts. While this is something we thrive on when engaging with media, what does this say for young people, for all gay people, when the relationships they see are doomed to failure or for one of the gay characters to die? To simply be a moment of conflict, something intense, only to fizzle out in despair, death and the inability to be together. *Brokeback Mountain, Moonlight, Call Me by Your Name* are some of the most successful gay films to be on the big screen over the past few decades. How many of them feature a happy ending? None.

Films, books and TV help to change perceptions, they reflect ourselves, they reaffirm who we are. If the message that we receive is purely that a same-gender relationship can't succeed, what does that do to the insecurities, the belief that we don't deserve a healthy relationship, the perception of the world of the queer community? It's fundamental that we ask: what does the daily consumption of media stereotypes do to us internally and externally?

While, indeed, life and especially that of a gay person shouldn't be sugar-coated, shouldn't we have examples where a gay relationship succeeds? What message are we as a community receiving when all we see is love that cannot survive? What sign of hope does a working-class queer person receive when the depictions of themselves only reaffirm what the world thinks?

There are schools of thought, such as Social Learning Theory, that believe as humans we develop behaviours and knowledge through mimicry and observation. If we apply that to a lifetime of either being exposed to no or negative representation, then we may begin to adopt what we observe, read and consume as our ways of being. When we live in a dominant heteronormative society with so many of us not even knowing any other queer people, especially when growing up, the place we go to learn our social cues, behaviour and culture is the media. I lived out what I saw and read and knew to be true. I felt no self-worth so I carved out what I felt I deserved in the love I received from others and for myself. I've lived with continuous mental health problems, seen my life as disposable. The damage from negative representation can be unquantifiable.

As people, we are inclined to engage and connect with what reinforces our world and what we know, to connect with established and preordained categories. As such, living in a world where the white, middle-class heteronormative is the dominant and majority culture explains why this is what is so often depicted in the arts. They portray what they know, or assume, and it's not often the truth of people coming from minorities. Think of the egregious characters from the 1990s – Will and Jack from *Will & Grace*, Tom from *Gimme Gimme Gimme*, who play into the tired caricatures of 'passing' or effeminate.

It is also down to the fact that so many of those industries have a distinct lack of people at the table who are people of colour, queer, disabled and working class. The Creative Industries Policy and Evidence Centre reports that in 2019, 16 per cent of people from working-class backgrounds worked in the creative industries,[3] a decrease of 1.4 per cent since 2014. According to a 2020 survey by the Publishers Association, 11 per cent of the UK publishing workforce are LGBT+, 8 per cent are people with a disability and 13 per cent are from BAME backgrounds, but there was no data on people from working-class backgrounds.[4] Minorities remain a minority. If the category isn't collected, working-classness will remain invisible, and so too will other intersections.

When there aren't those voices at the table, the world will continue to reflect what is known and understood by dominant cultures and people. They control what we see, shape how we view ourselves and others. What we see is a mirror of their lives, concerns, perspectives and not ours. Trans people depicted as predators or murderers, lesbians minimised and eroticised for the heterosexual gaze, bisexuals erased or depicted as greedy. These tropes are so dominant and damaging and highlight how little true and positive representation there is in creative industries.

Queer characters on screen have increased since the 1990s, where they were few and far between and nothing more than stereotypes, and the importance of this representation for our well-being and acceptance can't be understated. We also need to question the way we are depicted, both as working-class and as queer, and even beyond monogamy. We need representation, and the fight for this continues, but we also need positive representation. As a child I longed to see someone reflect my reality and to give confirmation that what I was feeling was normal. But what impact do these tropes of gay relationships that cannot last do? So many same-gender relationships that we're presented within literature, media and culture are unhealthy, damaging and are destined to doom or death.

Series like *Queer Eye*, a show where five queer presenters help to positively transform lives, and *Schitt's Creek*, which follows a family that loses their fortune where the son, David, is gay, and the normality the show promotes around sexuality, shows us the love, happiness and positivity that can happen either in relationships or as a community. *God's Own Country*, set in Yorkshire with a sheep farmer, Johnny, and a Romanian migrant worker, Gheorghe, follows the love story of two working-class men. Even though there is conflict in their story, it still manages to end in happiness. Newer shows such as *It's a Sin*, set during the emerging HIV crisis in the 1980s, or *Heartstopper*, based on a group of friends beginning to understand their sexuality and gender in secondary school, both depict serious and traumatic events but also show the power of community, friendship and family. They show relationships that are healthy, depictions of queer people from all classes and races without being entirely dependent on tropes.

This is the type of inclusion and representation that needs to be the standard for queer people to view themselves better and to overcome the stigma and low self-esteem we're conditioned to have. Increasing stories from minorities helps to demarginalise them. Every person needs and deserves to have their own world confirmed. That is why the arts are so important as we can participate in those people's lives and have our own validated. When all I saw growing up was nothing at all or negative, unhealthy and stereotyped representations, it reinforced what I had been taught as a child: I was wrong, I won't find love, I won't be happy. Many of these remain in what we consume today.

Boosting these stories can help them flourish in real life, find acceptance by people who don't inhabit the minority borders. The author of *Giovanni's Room*, James Baldwin, himself stated that the story is about 'what happens if you are so afraid that you finally cannot love anybody'.[5] This is the scenario for so many queer people. Not only are we afraid that our love won't be accepted by society, family and friends, but we're afraid that we don't deserve that love, or that it can't actually exist.

Every date, every relationship – no matter how strong the bond, the connection, the desire – there was an expiry date. I had a lifetime of being rejected for who I am, not having validation that I was normal, not knowing that it was possible to be with another man due to the law and society's stigmas. When the films and books we use to escape reinforce those doomed narratives, is there any surprise that at some point we give up dreaming and believe it's all we deserve? I destroyed love because I couldn't find it for myself. Difference is born on the lips. It's replicated and mass produced, too.

There have been nights where I have cried as I tried to sleep after a failed date, a hook-up, a relationship that had gone past its use-by date. Wishing and wondering why it wouldn't last, why they wouldn't stay, just a little longer. Is it any wonder why I, and other queer people, feel like we don't deserve more than a fleeting moment, an unhealthy relationship, an abusive relationship, a relationship that's doomed, when that's the image we're shown? We will hurt each other, hurt ourselves, destroy things, destroy ourselves, self-destruct and destruct together because that's what we've been taught. It's one of the few narratives we've been given. We look for the love we think we know and deserve. We beget the love we receive. So many of us faced rejection and hatred towards our sexuality growing up so we repeat that in adulthood through patterns of rejection and destruction. We seek out validation and love even for a moment, even in the unhealthiest of ways, because that is what we have been shown, and to fill the void we lacked when we were growing up. We aren't incapable of love; we find it difficult to accept it.

We always have to choose between history and love. That is our real dichotomy. History always seemed to win. History is written by the winner. So many of our art forms give power to this history, consign us to history, a heterosexual history, a heterosexual story, a heterosexual lens. This is not to say healthy, queer relationships don't exist, they do in abundance. This is not to say that queer people can't find happiness, we can. But our art forms need to take accountability in how we are represented. Not just for how we perceive ourselves, but how the rest of the world does, too. Let us write and paint and sing and film a queer future away from the past that has been given to us. We deserve a life and a love not predetermined by the constraints and damage done to us by a hetero society.

The constant negative portrayal of queer people, their relationships and the working class inhibits our ability to love ourselves and others when we replicate hateful and heteronormative structures within our own community. While we are gaining more representation, and this fight needs to continue, we also need positive and healthy depictions of same-gender love, relationships and people. Queer people are not homogenous and should not be depicted dichotomously nor shamed for not looking or acting like an idealised heterosexual man. We need to celebrate our diversity, differences and how we present our gender and sexuality in a variety of beautiful ways.

Chapter Four

I stared at the mirror behind the bar. Trying to find my reflection behind the spirit bottles. The dark figure staring back. Soaked in red and pink and blue lights. There for a minute, then plunged back into shadow. The room hummed with sweat and perfume and testosterone. My feet sticking to the pools of sickly coloured drinks. I sucked in my cheeks to try to make my cheekbones more prominent. Pulled my neck up so my jawline was more pronounced.

I tugged at my t-shirt, worried it didn't fit well enough, or that it fitted too well, whether I looked overweight, too muscular, not muscular enough. I shuffled, worried about what others thought, catching their eye and looking away. Crossing my arms over my chest to try to hide away my body in case it wasn't good enough. Trying to push away the thoughts that my body was inadequate and enjoy the thrum of the pop music vibrating through the room. The bodies writhing, the shrieks and laughter. The image in the mirror didn't reflect what was there in the flesh.

Whether on a date or out with friends I'd always had this lingering anxiety about how my body looked. A consuming worry that I was overweight or not muscular enough, much of my confidence relied on whether I felt physically good enough. The body insecurities didn't begin in my adulthood but in my adolescence, in an attempt to appear more heterosexual and masculine as my body changed from preteen gymnast to teenage gymnastic drop-out, which culminated in muscle dysmorphia. Muscle dysmorphia, a type of body dysmorphia, is where a person views their body as weak or insufficiently muscular despite what may be the reality. Growing up in the 1990s, the male celebrities and icons in the media exhibited a more muscular frame, think Brad Pitt and Leonardo DiCaprio. These were our standard, the ultimate men we should aspire to be that optimised the gender norms and codes that were instilled in us as children.

As a kid, the toilet was my Narnia. The place I could step into, lock the door and escape the outside world. Inside, new worlds opened up and formed in my head or on the pages of a book. My legs swinging as I sat reading *Horrible Histories* or a book on myths or Roald Dahl. I'd read the TV magazine and what was on that week, eyes flitting over TV and film stars and their chiselled jaws, flawless skin and coiffed hair. I flipped through clothes catalogues and linger longer on the underwear section. My eyes drawn there, unable to break away, despite the fear, despite the heat in my cheeks.

Growing up, I never had a mirror in my room, I hated looking in them, and still don't sleep with one in my room. I was scared of mirrors because of what they would reveal. We look in mirrors to hunt ourselves. We look in mirrors to connect the two dislocated parts of our selves: the interior and exterior that never meet, which never match up. Something inside, and outside, made me feel that I wasn't right. Everything around me was geared up to assert that I had to like girls, women. I had to look and behave a certain way. Guys didn't like guys sexually or romantically.

The kids on the estate and in primary school made me know that it was wrong from their homophobic taunts or by making fun of me for doing 'girls' activities'. They were all the typical boys who strutted around, playing football, chasing after girls. There was a type of masculinity, a physicality they adhered to. They rooted shame into who I was and asserted that there was a type of masculinity I had to aspire to if I wanted to be accepted into the club. It was one where clothes were covered in oil and grease, dirt and white paint from football pitches. The gaze of others is so important to queer people growing up – are we performing our gender expression 'properly', are we physically being feminine or masculine as we ought to be?

From watching them, I learned what masculine was and how I should behave and how my body should be. I mirrored heterosexual life and people because I had no exposure to anything else. We had parents, family, siblings, friends and others to learn from about how to be and mimic their behaviour. I knew no gay people, and the few instances of gay people on TV were caricatures. I emulated what I saw on the estate, the men I saw on TV, the men around me: heterosexual and muscular. As one study on body dysmorphia found, 'Appearance comparison was one of the strongest predictors of body dysmorphic disorder symptoms.'[1] I compared myself to them because physically they represented what I believed a man should be.

Becoming a teenager, I knew I wasn't going to allow myself to make the same mistakes I made as a kid. I was approaching my late teens and I wasn't in a long-term relationship like the other guys. Some of the kids on the estate, or guys at school, bragged about their new girl, who'd they'd had sex with. Most of them were probably exaggerating to try and get 'man points', but it only heightened my feeling of inadequacy knowing that I wasn't even close to fulfilling what I was supposed to as an apparent heterosexual man.

My friends at school had all been the rugby players, the ones that girls wanted to be with: tall, athletic, academic, undeniably straight. The men on TV, the sport stars, the models, people at school; it didn't matter where I looked, there was one type of masculinity: muscular bodies that symbolised strength and athleticism. There were very few other representations that were idealised in the same way in the mainstream. They all followed the script: get the girl, marry, have kids. The world I lived in had space only for homogeneous masculinity, which came with the prerequisite of being straight. There was little, more often no, representation of queer people.

As teenagers, we are no longer expected to show that we identify as boys but instead have to display and actualise that we are now living up to what a 'man should do'. Teenagers utilise this opportunity to assert dominance and their own masculinity, thus rejecting homosexuality, by mocking other males who do not display these qualities in the way that is expected. *Balls dropped yet? Bet you're a virgin. He speaks like a girl. How many you had? He looks like a weed.* These were the kinds of statements and questions thrown about at school, all to denote whether we were validating our masculinity through sex, our physical prowess and heterosexuality.

It's a way to ensure that we aren't viewed as feminine and gay, to make sure we adhere to the heterosexual matrix. Moving from childhood, the gender signifiers of boy morph into those of man: the deepness of our voices, the ability to grow a beard, our virility, or ability to attract women. It evolves into how well we perform the heterosexual narrative. The foundations of what constitutes masculine and how to perform it is learned in childhood, passed from generation to generation, adapting with society and environment. I was surrounded and brought up by strong women who influenced who I was; I could never reconcile myself with a dichotomy where the feminine was viewed as weak. If we stray from the script, we are taught shame and are rejected. Deviation risks being seen as different.

It'd been years since I was a kid on the swing, on top of the slide, leaning over backwards and upside down on the climbing frame watching the teenagers play football. The curve of a back as they leaned into kicking the ball. Leaned into the girls and kissed them. Leaned into going from boy to man. I had asked to get an ear piercing like them, have the curtains boy-band haircut they all seemed to sport. They did it so effortlessly, like it all came naturally to them. I came to learn what they sweated and breathed so easily was masculinity. They all moved so seamlessly from boyhood to manhood, I never seemed to make it there. Even though I was now the same age as they were, I didn't feel like I'd stepped into the skin marked with man.

To survive we metamorphosise into what is viewed as acceptable. What was acceptable was athletic and muscular as that's what the world told me meant heterosexual, what a real man was. That was the only vision of masculinity that I had, so I replicated it. The body is a vessel for masculinity. I was terrified to admit that I was gay. It was against everything I knew to be right. I hid my sexuality behind sport and exercise because that was the image I could control when people looked at me. They wouldn't have seen effeminate, they wouldn't have seen gay, they wouldn't have seen the poof who tumbled across the green. I hid my true self and, in its place, developed muscle dysmorphia.

I found myself noticing guys in a way that was different to before. Someone had scrawled 'Mike Handrick is gay' in big red letters on a desk because he thought I fancied his girlfriend. Gay was used to tarnish me as there was no worse thing at school. The seal was breaking. It was all starting to seep out. What I had tried to hide wasn't working. I could feel my eyes drawn to guys on the street when I hadn't before. I was constantly probed about why I hadn't had a proper girlfriend yet, causing anxiety attacks. People were worried. I was paranoid everyone could see what I was trying to hide. So many kids at school were bullied for being weak, skinny, unathletic, for deviating from the male ideal. *Sissy, weak, poof, weird.* I'd learned my lesson from childhood and wouldn't be tricked twice. I had to stopper it up: seal away the gay. It had all begun with trying to be fitter so I could play lacrosse better.

The drip of sweat, the grind of muscle, the thump of weights hitting the floor. Grunts and sighs, panting. The music blaring, veins popping under skin stretched too tight. Nike and Adidas stepped by me. I could smell them, see the drip of sweat on their legs, the throb of testosterone. The laughter and slaps on the back, slaps of flesh. My own body twitched on the floor. I stared around, hoping someone would stop by and check if I was okay. No one offered me a hand, no time to spare when youth and strength have an expiry date. I scraped myself up, fell to the floor again. Every sinew burned, my legs searing, the pain making me gasp and tear up. The lactic acid had built up so much, my legs so tight from overexercising that I could no longer support myself.

I lay there watching everyone exercise. Masculinity could be wrung out from their tops. The peacocking, the clenching of biceps and staring at multiple reflections staring back at them, the sly glances at other guys to see who was outperforming them. The swirl of protein shakes, frothing mouths, the collective eyes checking out women. I was just as strong and muscular as them yet I was still terrified, still didn't feel like I was like them. They were part of the 'heterosexual club' I didn't belong to. It was their space, a man's space.

When the strength came back to my legs, I hobbled to the scales. The red line quivering mockingly as I lifted myself onto it. Staring down, hoping for one more pound lost, another pound of muscle gained. Nine stone. Still more to lose, more to gain. I changed into my swimming shorts and swam for thirty minutes as per my routine. An hour and a half of cardio, an hour and half of weights, followed by swimming to wash it all off. Back in the changing room, towel-wrapped men strutted around, sweat and water beaded across muscle. I kept my eyes firmly fixed on the floor. Not letting my eyes drip over them, stopping myself from imagining what was outlined by those cheap, white towels. Too scared of someone thinking that my eyes were lingering, potentially locking eyes with someone else who recognised something in me that I didn't want to see in myself.

I pulled on an American Eagle polo shirt, stuffed my gym clothes into my lacrosse bag. My hands shook as I sat on the bus home from town. Not from the amount of training I had done but the fear that I hadn't done enough. After schoolwork and dinner, I'd go to my room and do it all over again. Using my brother's bench press, rounds and rounds of press-ups, sit-ups and crunches. My body fat percentage was around 10 per cent, yet when I looked at myself, all I saw was fat. I didn't see the six pack and the pecs. I looked in the mirror and it reflected what I saw and felt inside: monstrous. In the mirror, I pulled at the skin on my stomach, sucked in my cheeks. Twisted, turned, inspected, prodded, sighed. I looked in the mirror and someone else stared back at me. Overweight, useless, not fit enough, not muscular enough, not pushing hard enough. No pain, no gain. Not man enough.

To look at me you would have said otherwise. I had the 'V' body shape some guys aspire to, what the media told us to aspire to. You could trace the splits and canyons of my body, the sinew and the tendons. Every day, I'd do at least three hours at the gym, lacrosse training on Tuesdays for over two hours, matches and conditioning Saturdays for over two hours, then exercising at home to top it off. It was all followed by anxiety attacks as I felt it still wasn't enough.

Lacrosse was aggressive and physical; it wouldn't be seen as gay like gymnastics was. It – I – never felt enough. Not man enough, not straight enough, not strong enough, not clever enough, not rich enough, not good-looking enough. I understood the figures of the weight I was losing and the muscle I was gaining but they didn't compute in my head. No matter how many hours I did a day, no matter how much weight I was losing, how much muscle I was gaining, I didn't feel like I belonged to the man club, nor could I see it.

I hammered and chiselled and sculpted and moulded until an Adonis-like husk stood in front of me. I stepped into it, pressed my lips against it and breathed to give it life. There were no flaws, it was the perfect body. I walked through a house of mirrors and every reflection staring back was the ultimate representation of straight masculinity. No one saw or heard the person banging on the glass to get out. Something inside had slipped away from the blueprint so at least I could convince them otherwise on the outside. I sculpted my body so I could be similar to them, and knew that I would never be similar to them.

My pursuit to emulate this body type was partially driven to align more with the masculine rather than the stereotypes associated with effeminacy. I wasn't driven to have the body I had to attract women or anyone, but to fit in, to be 'one of the guys'. My obsession with exercising and having a 'perfect' body was driven by my own internalised homophobia and fear that by being associated as effeminate or weak would mean people could recognise that I was gay. Reports show that men with muscle dysmorphia are much more likely to adhere to masculine than female norms[2] and suffer from low self-esteem.[3] I adhered to the heterosexual and masculine norms more than I would have done to try to trick everyone – and myself – that I wasn't gay. My pursuit of being normal led me to try and live it out through my body.

Perhaps that is why, no longer a boy, I started to gaze so much at my reflection: because of that dichotomy between who I was inside and who I was expected to be outside. It became a way to validate whether or not I was physically performing masculinity in the expected way. I tried to catch glimpses of myself in every surface: a wing mirror, a window, a piece of cutlery. I looked to try to align, to make sure I wasn't something inferior on the outside. I shook and panicked and constantly thought that I had to do more. To be a man.

I felt that the world would reject my internal, true self whereas my physical self couldn't be rejected if I appeared muscular and masculine. By reaching physical perfection, I could be accepted when I couldn't accept myself. I believed it gave me power and control while I was trying to grapple with the inner turmoil of understanding my sexuality with nothing to validate or understand it. Yet, I didn't know that the effort to control everything would then consume me in turn.

My time at secondary school was filled with hollow kisses tinged with beer and regret. I lived in a meaningless body where validation came from how I looked and whether my body was acceptable to the gaze of the heterosexual world. Trapped in a statue that people thought was beautiful, but I thought was monstrous. The person within was monstrous. I was an imposter in a world where every day I pulled out a new skin from my cupboard to dress up as some middle-class boy, where a voice of someone else escaped my lips. I was an imposter in my own body wishing for a world, a time, a space where just for a night, just for a moment, I could be away from my own reality, where who I was and where I came from didn't matter.

I started to find ways to secretly indulge those fantasies, to find a new life in virtual reality. Down bandwidths and data instead of the glossy pages of a catalogue. Being gay wasn't a possibility or reality so I lived it out secretly. Forbidden fantasies were lived out through porn. Porn was my real introduction to being gay. I didn't know what was involved, how to do it. The browsing history was always cleared, retyping the URL to make sure it didn't appear. There are many who are alone and have no encounters with other gay people in reality or the media until later in life, thus porn can be their first encounter with the image of being gay, of understanding they're normal. From what we're exposed to, we learn from.

The stars in mainstream porn were exactly like the super heroes and athletes and actors on TV: ripped, rugged and handsome. They were all cookie-cut from the same mesomorphic dough and pumped up into replicas. This was my sole vision of homosexuality: gay but white, hyperstraight. I didn't see any other visions of homosexuality, how their body types and expression was any different to the straight world. While porn, for some, is about fantasy and extremes of desirability, our desires aren't homogenous, just like our bodies and gender expression. I found this image of masculinity no more concentrated than in the image of the working-class man: hyper-sexual, aggressive, dangerous.

The lad or chav becomes and 'remains an object – before, during and after his use – of disgust, filth and repudiation'.[4] Through consumption – via porn or reality – it conjures the gay man's own internalised sense of shame and worthlessness. Working-class gay men embody that internalised self-hate because they are viewed as the dregs of society while also bolstering the middle-class man's straightness by sleeping with someone who is perceived to be straight and aggressive. It also asserts a hierarchy within a minority of the middle-class gay man as superior to the working class to overcome this sense of shame that has been instilled from childhood bullying. This was what was expected of a working-class gay guy, what others wanted us to be. I didn't see myself like that, but on the streets and all around me I was being told that I had to be hypermasculine, transgressive.

For some, the working-class gay man is but a tool for the middle class to boost their sense of value and find an illicit moment with someone deemed as dangerous. Much of the working-class, or 'scally', porn takes this to the extreme where the scenes are often rape-like. There are issues of domina-tion and power dynamics here where gender, sexuality and class play into roles of dominating and submitting, and exhibiting prowess through that. We're viewed as an exaggerated depiction of masculinity to overcome internalised homophobia and misogyny. This depiction is dangerous and unhealthy. It reinforces what society has already deemed us, showing us that we are not people who are intelligent and passionate and caring, but a stereotype. The guys I knew on the estate would not have behaved like that; it is merely a caricature.

I found there to be a small amount of irony, now being an out adult, seeing the aesthetics of the working-class man becoming a trend within the gay community. I was called a townie and a chav for wearing tracksuit bot-toms; it was an image I was made to feel self-conscious about, one that on the estate would never be correlated with being gay. But in the late 2000s, hoodies, caps, tracksuits and trainers became assimilated and popularised by certain groups within the gay community. The stereotype of working-class men as hypersexual, aggressive and, above all, heterosexual, has been adopted to further present the image of being 'straight passing'. The clothing becomes a costume to present an image of hegemonic heterosexuality, presenting a masculine identity that allows someone to pass off as straight, an image that society can accept. It is a direct attempt to erase the feminine and shame that has been correlated with being gay since childhood and to present a more heterosexual front. We were taught a 'feminine man' was wrong and as such having sex with one whose gender expression is more feminine reignites that childhood shame and conditioning.

Being gay is a rejection of the male signifiers, rules and paradigms established to us as children. The commodification and festishisation of the working-class man are found in these roots. Being gay has historically been linked to the feminine and thus tied up with homophobia and misogyny. At its core, this working-class representation of the gay man is the epitome of hegemonic heterosexual masculinity. It's a reflection of wanting to present as hegemonically homosexual in response to the shaming and bullying we dealt with as children for not meeting those expectations. The feminine was set up as the antithesis.

As gay men, we 'seek ways to compensate for perceptions that [we] are less masculine'.[5] Throwing myself into sport, and its subsequent morph into muscle dysmorphia, was used as a shield to avoid any prejudice or discrimination for being anything less than heterosexual. I was consumed by paranoia, convinced that people thought I was gay, and I lived constantly with the threat that I could be found out somehow. The world, and media, had taught me that there was one vision for masculinity, which meant muscular and heterosexual, so I emulated that. I had always felt different, been told I was different, and so couldn't align with the gender identity I was told I had and should have. It made me try to align myself more with those around me, the boys on the council estate, the cool kids at school, to try to attain those masculine ideals.

'Minority stress', which is linked to discrimination and victimisation, also includes the internalised shame towards sexuality and can be linked to overall negative feelings towards the body and muscular dissatisfaction.[6]

Indeed, research supports this in finding that, overall, homosexual men have a greater body dissatisfaction than heterosexual men.[7] This can be linked to a variety of reasons from the oversexualisation of gay men and greater focus on the body in the media, through to the shame of not being heterosexual. We live in a society dominated by a hypermasculine physical depiction and shame for those who deviate from that standard.

These expectations filter down through to the gay community. For a long time, homosexuality was classified as an illness. The emergence of HIV and AIDS, and the subsequent epidemic, decimated and scarred the gay community. It left men debilitated and emaciated, the whole community traumatised by this unknown disease compounded by the abandonment and vilification that they received from government, the media and the wider public. Combined with the long-standing stereotypes of gay men as camp, effeminate and frail, gay men were facing unprecedented attacks for their sexuality. As a result, there has been an amplified view of gay men's physicality being linked to fragility and illness.

It creates a toxic pressure, from the media and from parts of the community, to reject weakness, illness and femininity, and replicate what is deemed normal: homogenous, hegemonic, heterosexual. The holy trinity. This translates into the gay world from porn, the development of the 'Tom of Finland' aesthetic, the media through to art. Artists like Rotimi Fani-Kayode and Robert Mapplethorpe were leading gay figures in the 1980s. Their work was genius, subversive, challenging. Mapplethorpe photographed women bodybuilders and confronted traditional notions of femininity, while his self-portraits brought fetish culture to the fore, and his portraits of men reflected and challenged the hypermuscular ideal of masculinity. The men are overtly muscular. Each one is reminiscent of an ancient Greek statue. Still, statuesque. They are the epitome of health and youth, which so starkly juxtaposes the bodies of gay men that were being stripped of both during the height of the AIDS epidemic, and the same virus Mapplethorpe was living with, while at the same time reaffirming the unrealistic expectations that society imposes on men to have this type of masculinity.

While today we do have more visibility and acceptance of body variety and gender from non-binary celebrities to the rise of drag culture subverting gender norms, we are still very much dominated by this hypermasculine and muscular being, whether on the screen, in porn or magazines, as the stalwart for what we should strive to be like. Without any irony that this idealised figure harks back to the homoeroticism found in antiquity. In fact, research finds that gay men are more likely to internalise this image and cause negative effects when feeling pressured to replicate what both heterosexual and gay media are pushing on us.[8] It highlights how we are subject to an appearance-focused culture that has a greater amount of sexual objectification,[9] nudity and focus on the body.[10] This representation is unhealthy and narrow. It is cis, white, heterosexual and ableist. There is no room for other versions of beauty, there is no spectrum. Different representations of larger men, race, disability and neurodiversity are rare. What room is there for other expressions of being gay? We need to interrogate and break down how this amplified vision of white gay masculinity with its corresponding structures and idealisms directly repress and ostracise other minorities and intersections as well as promoting misogyny.

Scroll through social media and it will be dominated by men posting pictures topless, at the gym, tensing every muscle and sinew in their body. Our bodies are the vessels for masculinity and if we can gain the validity for our bodies, our physical heteronormativity, we can gain validity for our sexuality that doesn't deviate, which isn't queer. If our bodies are heterosexual then it's okay to be gay. We're not poofs or femme or queer. We're real men despite loving men. Open up Grindr or any other dating app and it is littered with references to this. *Masc4masc, no femmes, no queers, straight-passing, butch, only real men.* Racism is rife, men are shamed for being bottoms, for being 'fem' as a direct link to this internalised homophobia and misogyny.

Both refute what it means to be a 'man' and being confronted with it means we have to acknowledge our own sexuality and our deviation from the heteronormative narrative that has been laid out for us. From the gender norms we are conditioned with in childhood and what is deemed masculine, the desire for a particular type of masculinity that is deemed as 'more straight' becomes entangled in how some gay men view and treat others. It directly feeds into why there is so much fem-shaming within the gay community. It makes a man confront his own sexuality and evokes the negativity, shame and hate we were conditioned to have towards it.

This concept of 'real man' pervades our community, it lingers over all of us, making us feel ashamed for not living up to this notion that we were conditioned to be like as boys, how media and others expect us to be as adults. We then replicate that shame within our own community: holding up the queer community to heteronormative ideals and standards.

Do we pursue physical perfection because we were conditioned to believe we were imperfect? We need to project a perfect physical representation of masculinity, which we didn't feel we had. Other people's gaze from childhood formulates our bodies and shapes our perspective of our own selves. Are we being too feminine, masculine, are we performing our gender correctly, are we muscular enough? Our bodies are a way to take control over something that we don't have. All of these pressures, exposure, conditioning are the formulation of becoming a man; we are born as a canvas, our gender is painted on it by society. By shifting the gaze of others, we can control what they think, thus how we feel. To survive we metamorphosise into what is viewed as acceptable.

The hegemonic masculine homosexual is a depiction to reassure heterosexual society that we aren't a threat. A caricature that won't disrupt or destroy their hierarchies, structures and values. If we're masculine in their way, it's safe as we're not breaking masculine norms. Just as the overly effete and camp homosexual depiction is a way to reassure straight people that we won't steal their women, that we can't attack or destroy or break their masculinity. There is also research that confirms that gay men 'experience a greater drive for thinness'.[11] By forcing gay men into this dichotomy of Adonis versus ephebe or twink, masculine versus feminine, heterosexual men can remain secure in their masculinity while in turn creating hierarchies of 'gayness' in our own community. The pressures we face as gay men to live up to one of these depictions as either camp or straight-passing directly links to body dissatisfaction, depression, anxiety, stress, eating disorders, muscle dysmorphia, shame, inadequacy, substance abuse and even suicide.

As a result, this can lead to someone becoming vulnerable in a relationship or to abuse due to feeling inadequate, ashamed or wrong. It creates a power imbalance, the need to receive validation for who you are from someone else rather than from yourself. Not feeling good enough can create a power and control imbalance if that insecurity is wielded by someone else. Being told you're not man enough, too feminine, too big, not muscular enough, not good enough can set off a spiral of needing that validation even when it comes from unhealthy sources.

I emulated the standard of male beauty and aesthetic from antiquity, the pin-up of our society's idealised male form. I perfected this physical manifestation of male beauty and masculinity. I replicated what was deemed as desirable, what society expects from a man. From the conditioning we receive as children, our musculature and strength are representative of being a real, heterosexual man. However, I replicated this ideal not knowing that it would also be perpetuated in gay culture.

These same pressures and expectations are found there too, lurking and blooming in different ways, tied up in toxic masculine ideals. So many of us have been shamed online or in person for our bodies, how we look or behave. We should be able to express our sexuality and gender free of pressures of societal expectation, not imposing and replicating it. We replicate this hate and expectation that comes from heterosexual masculine structures and weaponise it against each other when we should be supporting each other, embracing our differences and celebrating our expressions.

We find ourselves displaced in a culture that we can't see ourselves in nor belong to. The hate and shame and rage that is directed at us, is then rebounded at each other. Those who deviate from the white ideal – Eurocentric notions of beauty – those who deviate from the muscular. We create boxes and labels to form a community and ostracise those who don't fit it. We're rejected for our sexuality so body insecurity and obsession are a way to find validation and acceptance. We are made to feel uncomfortable, like we don't belong in our bodies, not only for how society sets up unrealistic expectations of the male form but also for our sexuality. A constant reminder that we are not heterosexual.

In the club, weaving my way through the crowd, drinking in the air and singing at the top of my lungs I stopped caring. I danced with my friends, trying to enjoy myself and the moment rather than what I thought of myself, my body or what others thought of it. Of course, the lingering insecurities and doubts are still there. When out or on a date, or even on a day-to-day basis, the body dysmorphia still lingers, but it isn't as destructive as it was.

It took me a number of years to start to love my body again, to understand that it shouldn't be defined by notions of gender or masculinity, but instead by whether or not I'm happy in it. I had to understand that I was living out a narrative that wasn't mine. Once I became happier in who I was, in my sexuality, it helped me unravel the dichotomy I felt. I'm no longer trying to be someone I'm not. I can express myself, my gender, my sexuality in the way I want to rather than how I believe society or others expect me to.

As a community, our strength, our beauty, comes from our difference. We defy the binary and heteronormativity. We disrupt the status quo. We have so many subcultures. Yet even within our own community, let alone society, we are pushed into believing that the binary and the hegemonic expression of masculinity is the acceptable way of being gay. Our media, both heterosexual and queer, need to step up and start showing greater body and gender representation to show beauty and masculinity beyond the mainstream. From our childhood, our carers and teachers need to stop using gender norms to box children into constrictive binaries where if they deviate from what is expected of a girl or boy they are wrong.

This isn't about shaming or condemning exercise and being proud of your body, far from it. Exercise plays an integral part in physical, mental and social well-being. I, and so many people, have felt its benefits. It can be transformative, healthy, lifesaving, confidence boosting. It's culture and society that corrupts it. We have to interrogate what constitutes 'man' and 'masculinity' and how each are compounded by societal expectations, gender norms around our physicality and sexuality, and how exercise can facilitate it. Breaking these down can help us to move forward so that we can stop applying unrealistic body pressures and gender norms to ourselves and replicating what heterosexual society expects of us.

We are negatively judged enough by society: we need to stop doing it to ourselves.

Chapter Five

Some believe that we are born into the world with an unwritten story. The waters breaking is the point where our narratives begin to flow. From our mothers' pain, we are given the chance to enter the world to make it our own. Our present is untouched by the past. We're yet to eat from the apple. To experience, to be influenced, to live, to fail, to love, to fall, to grow, have not yet been written on the blank pages that will eventually be filled with our life story. We are at chapter one: the moment we first breathe.

The route from water to air and flesh is treacherous. There are so many risks just to achieve that one momentous act. My umbilical cord was tied when my mum was in labour. My heartbeat dropped on the monitor every time there was a contraction. I was pulled and snipped and tugged into life. The umbilical cord severed. I was set free. Sharp air flowed into my lungs and filled them out, fluttering like the tiny chest of a bird. I opened my milky eyes and waited. For just a moment, the world is suspended. The pain endured for us to arrive is forgotten, and the pain that may come isn't even a thought.

Of all the souls, that soul chose to occupy my body and gave it the chance of life. An hour later, a different day, a different place there could have been no story being written now. Every second we live there could be another outcome, another life, another person. A kiss that doesn't happen, a job rejection, a cycling accident, a hand that isn't held, a caesarean that isn't

...1, a breath that isn't taken. Life isn't one clear-cut beginning, middle and end. Life is full of many beginnings and endings. Some last longer than others.

There is always a prologue that precedes chapter one. It's one we're not aware of but will influence us for the rest of our lives. Some may never be aware of it, some may never acknowledge it, some use it to their advantage, others will be tormented by it. We can't escape it. We come with an inheritance.

It's an inheritance from our parents, from their ancestors, a story that has been millennia in the making. A story that can destroy and give life, a story that can liberate and incarcerate. One with endless possibilities yet, for most, two distinct endings. It's entirely random how it's decided. Flip the coin, heads or tails? Two words: male and female. X meets X meets Y, sealed with an X. One letter, one variant results in two supposedly contrasting outcomes. One small letter shapes a life, an identity, expectation. It's one massive variant. It's all random, but when we are born so much is preordained. We are born with a story given to us without knowing.

'I carried you differently to your brothers,' my mum told me. She had carried my brothers lower so expected that I was going to be a girl. From the point parents know, or suspect, what sex their child is going to be, a million expectations, thoughts and considerations are made. From the name that will brand us with that sex, to the colour clothes and paint they will buy, to the journey our lives will take as we grow into adulthood. One child but two very different narratives.

Instead of a girl, I was the third boy. From birth we are sorted into 'male' and 'female' based on a doctor's assessment of our genitals and the assumption that our gender should reflect this. The sorting into the binary comes with the expectation that male and female will become two distinctly different people. Not being a girl shifted how I should be and how my life would unfold as society dictates. The world created around me and how I would be brought up would be starkly different, the way the world viewed me would be starkly different.

When we are born, and up until we start to be independent children, we need adults to make sense and order of the complexities and chaos around us. We put trust in the people who guide us through that, and put trust in the world they construct around us as true and infallible. It's not just essential activities such as eating, washing, walking and talking, but teaching us how to perform our assigned gender.

Our carers build up codes, behaviours, expectations and rules for us to navigate and understand how we should behave and perform our gender, which was inherited from theirs. This is crucial for our development and how to interact and function in the environment around us. It helps to build our role in society. Invariably, and unfortunately, our sex and gender play a significant part in defining the type of role we're given within these structures. There is an ideal image of how boys and girls should be, and how they should grow up to be, which is policed. This image has always been in flux and always faces challenges. The expectations during my childhood were a lot more stringent and less accepting of the relative fluidity there is now.

Since the 1990s, a lot of progress has been made in the perception, and representation, of sex and gender. There is greater visibility of gender fluidity and genders beyond the binary, which are challenging binary gender norms and becoming more accepted in the collective eye. Drag queens and kings, trans actors, artists and writers, and celebrities; male YouTube and TikTok stars give make-up tutorials, fashion houses make non-binary clothes. Writers and performers such as Shon Faye, Travis Alabanza, Kit Redstone and Paris Lees are all exposing systemic inequalities and showing the world what it means to be trans and live beyond the binary, which would have been inconceivable twenty years ago.

But we are still in need of both a systemic and a cultural shift in how children are raised respective to the binary. Before Western colonisation, many cultures had more than two genders, and some still do. Some societies around the world recognised more than five genders that include cisgender, transgender and androgynous. It was Western society that helped ship homophobic and gender-restrictive laws across the world, alongside the other atrocities that came with colonialism. Gender and sex ideals are fluid and on a spectrum. Everyone has their own expression; however, it is patriarchal Western society, culture and tradition that imposed only two distinct boxes: male and female.

As a boy I did not adhere to, nor meet, the unattainable vision of what it means to be 'male'. I didn't obey the rules of the game. I didn't mimic the aggressiveness and physicality of the other boys around me with the guns and cars that surrounded them. I rocked bright pink boots, played the witch or the fairy when we made up plays to perform and dreamed about being a mermaid in the froth and waves. I didn't match the blueprint set out for me.

We must have been still living in America, or visiting family there, as it's the only time I remember we were allowed McDonald's when we were young. We sat down with our Happy Meals and I rummaged inside the box to look for the toy. It was blue and red and shiny with four wheels, *Hot Wheels*. But I was disappointed. This wasn't the toy I had asked for at the counter. My parents said I could go ask to swap it, so I went back to see if I could have one of the dolls instead. The woman smiled at me, 'They're for girls.'

I was confused and hurt that I wasn't allowed one. At home I had dolls. I wasn't told to choose an Action Man or a gun or a car. Sometimes I would play with my brothers and their toys. But it happened that I preferred dolls, Care Bears and other childhood activities that – as I learned in that McDonald's – are so often only imagined as being for girls. I wrote stories in A3 pads and read books; I loved toys and activities where I could create new worlds, people and places. Consciously, at least, I don't think I was thinking about gender as I played or wrote or imagined. I never thought that I was doing anything strange, or that I wasn't a boy, nor did my family. It seemed there were bigger forces outside my door that did.

My cousin, Steph, and I were inseparable growing up. We had sleepovers most weekends where we read, watched films, and held the microwave popcorn bag on opposite sides to pull it open together and breathe in the buttery, salty steam. We stuck glowing stars to the ceiling and made blanket forts where we whispered our secrets, discussed our book ideas and made dream diaries.

When it was time to go back home, Steph would let me borrow one of her toys. I was never good at making decisions – I'm still not now – and she would do a countdown to help force me to choose. I'd flit between dolls and Polly Pocket and My Little Pony until I ran out of time and I had to just grab one to take with me. I would peep out of Steph's front door to check no one was around before I dashed home. I ran on the tips of my toes across the glass-spattered estate with a pink pony under my shirt. At corners, I checked down alleys for anyone who might spot my trinkets. The Happy Meal had taught me secrecy. I learned that toys and colours were loaded with meaning and danger.

Hiding wasn't something natural to me: my parents said I was a fearless child. I'd leap out from the tops of trees, be the first to go down the big hill on my bike, wander off by myself in airports and theme parks, then when I was found I wasn't scared at all. But then the name calling started, and started to get to me. The laughter, the stares, the names began from others who couldn't understand the smiling boy in pink boots holding a doll. *Where are your dollies? Why didn't they call you Michelle? Why aren't you a real boy?* The other children and adults seemed to instinctively know something wasn't right, but, of course, this wasn't an instinct they were born with – they had just learned faster than me.

Their eyes taunted, their laughter dripped into my ears until it forced me to learn that I had to have a private and public self. I was a fearless child until fear was put into me. I went from dressing as Baby Bop, fabulous and pink, for Halloween to being wrapped up in blues and reds and blacks. I withdrew into myself, made a refugee from my identity.

I had to adapt and evolve to survive. I'd say adapt in order to be accepted as one of them, but children's memories last a long time when they notice a difference, when one amongst their ranks has been branded as different. They don't forget or forgive a transgression, even if you try not to repeat it. My mum told me that she carried me differently; I soon learned that difference is a bad thing to most people. The creation of my fact and fiction selves had begun.

Through a series of rejection and validation, we begin to learn that as boys we must reject and denigrate feminine symbols and identity to assert and conform our manhood and for others to accept us as boys. We all grew up hearing pink was for girls, blue was for boys. In fact, pink, make-up, heels and flamboyant clothes were all deemed masculine, a symbol of power and wealth in different epochs. It's only in more recent history this has changed. Siri Hustvedt sums it up: 'Most boys in contemporary Western culture begin to resist objects, colors, and hairdos coded as feminine as soon as they have become certain of their sexual identity, around the age of three.'[1]

This is a direct result of the codes, signifiers and behaviour affirmation we receive from adults to ensure that our assigned gender 'matches' our sex. For boys to know they are displaying and performing masculinity correctly they need a standard to hold it up against, to know what is wrong. That is the female. We cannot be boys if we display characteristics, behaviours and interests that are correlated with the feminine. By continuously performing these masculine acts and roles it validates our gender and other people's belief of it.

I cried a lot when I was young. I cried when I fell over, I cried at films and books, I cried because I missed my family in America. I soon learned that this was a threat to my masculinity and acceptance to boyhood. *Don't be a girl. Sissy, wimp. Go play with the boys. That's not what boys do, don't you want to grow up and be a man?* Insults and conditioning, even beatings, are used to shame us not to deviate from the codes and signifiers that we have been taught. I was told to eat the crusts on my sandwiches as it would 'put hair on my chest'. We are taught to aspire to, and behave according to, an idealised hegemonic ideal of masculinity both physically and emotionally. This abuse is so commonly used to shame boys into stoicism as emotional displays are a clear violation of male gender codes. The expectations for men to be emotionally voiceless contribute to the higher suicide rates in men, particularly young men.[2]

From birth we enter into a world with 'heterosexual assumption',[3] in which we are forced to live out in heterosexual structures and narratives on the basis that we are all presumably heterosexual. From that very point on, the structures are built to lock us into that narrative and depict anyone who falls out of it as deviants, ostracised and treated different. Gender scripts, narrative in visual and written media, toys, language, clothes are all coded to ensure that we play into that assumption. My family accepted, supported and loved me for who I was, my interests, my differences without any questions. It was when I stepped out of the safety of my home that the world imposed those assumptions, those structures, those shackles.

Gender becomes a weapon, a tool, to ensure that a boy conforms and behaves according to a certain model of heterosexual masculinity while at the same time correlating the feminine as something negative and subordinate to masculine performance. In a survey of education practitioners, 64 per cent agreed that 'gendered assumptions affect boys' ability to talk about their emotions';[4] from the exposure they've had around them, what they've been taught, and what others, adults and other children, expect of them. From the earliest of ages, emotion is considered feminine and dangerous, yet not expressing emotion poses more danger.

Hustvedt further explains how in Western culture, 'the "feminine" has far more polluting power for a boy ... than the "masculine" for a girl'.[5] For example, a girl turning up to school in trousers is generally perceived as more acceptable than a boy in a dress. And this continues into adulthood: we've all heard that mainstream neoliberal feminist advice to women in business is to 'lean in', to behave more like men to get ahead. A boy breaking these gender signifiers and performing those behaviours traditionally associated with the female invokes the fear of the antithesis of established heterosexual dominant masculinity: homosexuality.

Effeminacy for centuries has been a signifier of homosexuality. By displaying more 'feminine' traits, a boy is seen to be breaking the narrative to grow up, marry and have children with a woman. Teaching boys that the feminine is negative and correlating it to homosexuality, we are brought up to see both as shameful and wrong. The root of homophobia finds itself in misogyny. In fact, 'much of the abuse and harassment' towards children who do not align with gender stereotypes, then as queer people in adulthood, 'stems from gender stereotypes'.[6]

The difference we are forced to feel as children breeds a sense of shame, a belief that we aren't normal compared with others around us that display a certain type of masculinity. Growing up with the fundamental belief that you are wrong because you don't meet an imposed, projected singular version of masculinity does untold damage mentally and psychologically. This is particularly damaging at an age where we begin to solidify our identities, and when that identity isn't validated, we carry that shame and self-hatred through to adulthood, in our relationships with others and ourselves.

Shame is debilitating, even more so when it is applied to your own identity, instilling a sense of worthlessness, lack of self-esteem and respect that can translate into mental health issues and power imbalances in relationships during adulthood. Many sources find that 'gender stereotypes create harms in terms of mental health long after childhood',[7] and that they 'cause specific harms to LGBT people in later life'.[8] I was forced to carry a stigma with me because of these social constructs. That bottle filled with a storm of emotions would shatter in adulthood.

Our early developmental years are a way to enforce that the binary of biological sex corresponds to two genders. We enter a world that assumes we're heterosexual and cisgender, and the narratives are built up around us to ensure we don't deviate from these. There is no room for a spectrum. It lays the foundation for what is expected from us as adults and as humans to ensure that we continue its reproduction, formulating two distinct groupings of breadwinner and homemaker. It constructs and perpetuates archaic systems of hierarchy and structure, which encourages misogyny and homophobia. It sets up the binaries of dominance and subservience, right and wrong that will be used to ostracise other people who deviate from expected roles and gender expression.

If we do not conform, we are inherently breaking how society is constructed, we are inherently wrong. Being othered and shamed from the youngest age can make you feel displaced in your own body for the rest of your life. Feeling different as you don't live up to the gender ideals laid out for you from birth. The shaming for not conforming to gender stereotypes is irrevocably linked to sexuality, and the heteronormative narrative will have a long-lasting impact on our mental health, making us feel we don't belong, we're not normal. The narrative that is given to us before birth is powerful and it's destructive long after we've survived the playground and the 'words that will never hurt me'.

Ever since I was a kid, I pushed myself into the pages of myth, folk and fairy tales. Curled up on the sofa or in bed, in the back of the car, or floating in the bath I memorised each story. I wished I could be like those characters and transform into something else to escape my own story. Metamorphosise into another person, a tree, an echo. There is a reason why I come back to myth and legends and fairy tales so much in my life, as they were my first love and influenced me more than I realised at the time. The darkness, the forests where shadows and danger lurked, witchcraft and spells and terrible endings for terrible children.

The narratives we are told, most often as kids, are sometimes the most influential of all. And, anyone who loves books knows that they are not merely words but have the power to influence. The other literary influence in my childhood came in the form of religion.

The pope has the Popemobile, we had a green Vauxhall Chevette nicknamed the Bogeymobile that drove us to redemption every Sunday. I'd be sat on a hard, wooden pew with my legs dangling over the edge and a copy of Bible stories for children in my hands, watching the rainbows from the stained-glass windows play out on the stone floor. Squished between my brothers, pulling at my collar, shuffling and snickering as we created nicknames for all the regulars. We slumped up and down from the pews dutifully to kneel and pledge our allegiance to the man hung up on a cross.

In tendrils of incense and the ache of my knees on the pews, prayer became a ritual to bury my true self, to be obedient to God's will and narrative for me. The same one that was expected of us all. One of the first things Christianity teaches you is that love is between a man and a woman. Being told that you'll be condemned to hell and brimstone as a child for loving someone of the same gender is, well, enough to put the fear of God into you. It's a terrifying image and one that lingers with you well into adulthood for simply loving another person. Christianity teaches that women were beget from men, and so were inferior, and that Adam and Eve were created to multiply. It was the woman who tempted humans into sin. These stories have sought to empower men and subordinate women and other minorities for two thousand years.

Religion is the foundation for the heteronormative narrative that controls and guides our societies and cultures in the West, even if many of us see ourselves as secular. Christianity developed into a political tool by Western churches and states dictating that we should get married, we must be monogamous, we must procreate – all tied to the heterosexual, all to weaken women in society, all to empower heterosexual men. This is despite some origin stories depicting powerful women or as one being, the hermaphrodite, which becomes weaker when they are divided into two genders. Christianity and Abrahamic religions formulate the foundations of patriarchal society and depict women as weaker. Each is filled with symbolism, deities and stories rife with male power and heteronormativity. Jesus died for us so we could be straight. It perpetuates and reinforces the structures, codes and expectations we are taught by family and friends, but with the caveat of eternal damnation. Perhaps it was apt that I was baptised in a white gown with ruffled sleeves.

Perhaps it was religion that inspired me to become a writer. The Bible was fantastical, it was dark, full of death and consequence. There were men swallowed by whales, a woman turned into a pillar of salt, the world flooded and trapped souls flung out onto the waves. What feels fictional, unreal, supernatural, can be fact. Jesus can raise the dead and turn water into wine, we were taught to be like Jesus, so surely, with enough faith, my own miracle of pretending to be someone else would be just as simple. Perhaps that is where I learned to fictionalise myself. All it takes is a story, a breeze from the lips to give it life and let it run its course. But I should have learned my lesson from the Bible that those stories can last and cause damage, and stories bound in the same book can so often contradict each other.

Fairy tales play an important role in the shaping of children's imaginations and their expectations of the world and themselves. They are literary gloves that are filled with a society and culture's view on gender, sexuality and roles according to the social code of a specific time. They're bestowed with new meaning to reflect conflicts, expectations and idealism. Fairy and folk tales are the first narratives that many children are exposed to, and so they play a specific and essential role in formulating and reinforcing the gender codes and structures that we're taught by our carers. They utilise a shared symbolic language that signifies idealised characteristics of the masculine and the feminine that we should emulate and replicate for our own roles in society.

Little Red Riding Hood, for example, reinforces the idea that girls shouldn't be curious. Girls should be subservient, obey the rules and not stray off the path otherwise they will be devoured by the wolf. The tale tells us that sexual exploration and virility should be restricted (only fuck one man, and only do that to have children), and that the little girl can only be validated, redeemed and saved by a man, the woodcutter. Women fall into one of two types: good and beautiful versus monstrous and wicked. Witches – women who digressed from this 'pure' narrative – must be killed for taking away the virginal princess. There is no deviation from this narrative: a woman can't be good as well as powerful and assertive, a man can't be feminine. Everything should be tied up nicely at the end with a marriage. These characters are archetypes for the roles we are conditioned to believe are the only way of living, and how our lives are destined to be. Princes and princesses have two distinct roles: one valorises and validates violence, physicality and stoicism; the other idealises servitude and subservience to the male. Story after story, there is really only one narrative, heterosexuality, which is only complete and successful with the unification of man and woman.

Think of all the Disney films – *The Little Mermaid, Snow White, Cinderella*: same story, same ending. Boys, be good, be manly, be strong and you'll be rewarded with the ultimate goal of marriage, wife and children. Girls, be obedient, docile and beautiful and you'll be rewarded with marriage, children and a man to save and validate you. From our earliest years we are exposed to the narrative of men being the breadwinners and women being the homemakers, a narrative itself so damaging in later life. In fairy tales, and in so much of the media we consume, there is no variety to the unrealistic and homogeneous types of gender we are presented. Children who do not see themselves reflected in these characters or tropes end up feeling alienated and alone. I did not see myself reflected in these characters. I did not see myself mirrored in the other children around me.

That's why I, and so many queer people, are drawn to the villains. Think of Ursula, the queer icon based on the drag queen Divine, who subliminally warns Ariel about the straight man: they'll make you voiceless, take your freedom and you'll only be 'fully human' when he chooses to kiss you. The bad guys who are often presented as flamboyant and camp – think Scar in *The Lion King*, Hades in *Hercules* – taught Generation X about the codes of homosexuality before we even really knew what that meant. In fact, modern retellings sanitise and heterosexualise the original tales that have so much fluidity, queerness and darker meanings.

The villains were forced to adapt and hide just like I had to. They inhabit a world that despises them, casting them to shadowed lairs and underground spaces. They – we – are forced to transform into what the dominant culture demands we should be like, or be destroyed for our refusal. Heterosexuality overcomes homosexuality, the virtuous and subservient get the guy over the lustful and assertive. In these fairy tale worlds, in the real heteronormative world, binaries become normalised, and dichotomies are used to put people in their place. How can one type of masculinity be validated and praised without vilifying a different type? There is evidence that young children who read storybooks that 'challenge gender stereotypes' can lead to 'positive outcomes in the wider world'.[9] Fairy tales have always been powerful, so often their power has been to restrict rather than to liberate.

Instead, I found love and freedom in complex women characters away from religion and the standard fairy tales for good children: witches, Medusa, the evil stepmother, goddesses. I was obsessed with shows like *Buffy the Vampire Slayer* and *Charmed*. With most shows about witches or vampire hunters, there is a coming out to the world or their circle of friends, just like with queer people. They are different, they keep secrets, powerful in their own way because they don't belong in the 'normal world'. Fundamentally, women and queer people are subversive. Perhaps, intrinsically, I noticed the way women were treated and so found comfort in women characters that wielded power and strength. It was a different power, one not drenched in the straight masculinity that I didn't identify with, one that I drew strength from. Yet, the world can't accept that strength, can't accept that difference.

The binary of male and female is the first that we're subject to and one that will dominate our lives. We use binaries and dichotomies to structure and organise the world around us so it functions. How can there be the concept of good if there is not the opposing force of evil? One must conquer the other – that is what we are taught from birth by the fairy tales we read. Binaries in effect regulate and impose hierarchies: good above evil, beautiful above ugly, light over dark, male conquers female, heterosexual eradicates homosexual. They are aspirational, inspirational, they give hope, they protect us, they erase us, they constrict us.

Yet it is this fundamental aspect of the binary that when utilised by humans becomes destructive. The binary is used to enforce dominance. This is seen throughout society in race, class, gender, sexuality and ability. There is always one that is asserted as better, normal, stronger. It sets one up as in opposition and inferior to the other. It is the binary of male and female that our world weaponises, uses to condition us, and is the benchmark to validate and judge us from infancy.

As boys, we are conditioned, whether intentionally or not, that the masculine is superior and the feminine is inferior, the other, and used as a derogatory force to teach and police male gender signifiers. The female, and the homosexual, are set up as the 'most threatening "other" of all'[10,11] because they challenge the hegemonic heterosexual masculine ideal that has been taught as right and omnipotent.

The rejection and shaming I faced, by the outside world, for not meeting gender norms, tried to mould me into a boy society expected. It forced me into a box I didn't belong in. Acceptance of who we are as children plays a pivotal role in our development, from our mental health to our self-esteem and how we view ourselves. The rejection of your gender expression and identity can cause a considerable amount of mental health damage. Validation is key in learning to love who we are, to feel normal and accepted by the people around us. The fearless child with no restraints was shackled and filled with insecurity and a lack of self-esteem. They made my body a prison.

So, I embodied those stories of transformation and concealment, trickery and deception that I loved so much. They taught me that you can change yourself, deceive others, but also that people aren't always what they seem. I just never expected to have to do so to survive. I became a real-life Loki – the trickster god, the one who metamorphosised, shifting gender and sexuality. He spun his being to his own whims. I was forced to wear a different skin, to adopt a way of being to survive that was unnatural to me. It taught me to correlate and associate being feminine and gay as bad and wrong, to be ashamed of who I really was. It was the point where I created a fact and fiction me.

Masculinity and femininity are not fixed. Gender – and sex – are not binary. We should not be forced to conform to paradigms and codes that are outdated, suffocating and restrictive. They are weaponised to shame children, to create hierarchies between male and female, hetero- and homosexual, cisgender and transgender. The damage the codes and rules we are taught are long lasting from misogyny, homophobia and transphobia, as well as the mental health issues that result from bullying, internalised self-hatred and shame. The fact that men are conditioned to view emotion as weak leads to the fact that 'men are less likely to seek treatment for mental health conditions',[12] and can be one contributing factor to the high levels of suicide in men. Cross-section that with being queer and the perfect mental health storm is created. It results in children, and adults, being ostracised and being told they're not normal for expressing their gender beyond what is socially accepted.

Change needs to come from education, from greater and wider representation in film, TV, art and books, as well as necessary legislation to recognise and protect people who do not identify as cis, male or female. Each child, every human, deserves to feel comfortable and safe in who they are. Every human deserves to feel worth, respect and that they are normal for however their gender is expressed. Across the world, there are thousands of varieties of masculinity, yet we are held up to the standard of one. We are socially conditioned into masculinity. All the pressures, exposure, expectations and shaming are the formulation of becoming a man.

From religion, to other children, from films, TV and books, we're conditioned to believe, and to perform, a masculine role that aligns itself with a homogeneous, heterosexual vision that if deviated from we are seen as other, feminine, gay. In places around the world, in different times, the combination of the feminine and the masculine in one body was revered. A symbiotic organism. We need to be more like that great primordial being, the hermaphrodite, we originate from. By splitting ourselves we are weaker. By forcing two distinct boxes, we are weaker. It directly affects our mental health, carrying the stigma, the feeling of being different or wrong into adulthood where this impacts our day-to-day life, as well as our relationships, where it can make us feel inadequate, creating a power imbalance.

Challenging gender stereotypes doesn't just need to come from the people who care for us as children, for them to teach us that we don't have to sit in two distinct boxes labelled 'male' and 'female'. Gendered language use can make such a difference in whether a child feels included or excluded in their environment and body. It needs to come from our education practitioners and the way they divide boys and girls, which not only affects a person's self-esteem throughout life but also their career choices. It needs to come from our books, where only five BAME characters feature in the top 100 children's books, LGBTQ+ characters are on the fringes, and gender stereotyping is still prevalent.[13] It comes from our industries that market and produce clothes and toys that perpetuate binary gender stereotypes, which is linked to girls feeling unable to do STEM subjects and the lower reading abilities of boys.[14]

It needs to come from our government and the Department of Education, curriculums, subject matter and what is being taught to children and the training given to practitioners about how to be inclusive. Change needs to come in our language and how we speak to children, and even adults, about their roles in society. We need to move beyond heterosexual assumption that controls so much of our lives, even before we are born, that affects us not only in adolescence but into adulthood. Challenging this narrative and its destructive potential can help move society away from restrictive views of gender and sexuality and reduce queerphobia, misogyny, and even suicide rates in men as adults.[15]

Years later, when I was older, I went through some boxes my mum had from my childhood. I found a letter I had written to my dad, who had stayed back in America to pack up the last of our stuff, in my dot-to-dot writing. It said how much I missed him, told him about our childhood dog, Freckles, and asked when my dolls would be arriving in England. My dad came back from America, but the dolls never arrived. The life I had being the boy who played with dolls was sealed up in a box somewhere in America with my name written on it. Never to be reopened and never to be seen again. Perhaps it was a warning, a metaphor, of sealing myself up.

Chapter Six

We spent nights reading *Sexing the Cherry* to each other. Him in Italian, me in English, learning the other's language where we twined imagery and worlds at the roots of our tongues. We read *Madame Bovary*, *Les Fleurs du mal*, Sartre. My mind unfurled and bloomed with language, darkness, emotion, possibilities that I hadn't found in books before, in a person before. We lived in languages we did not understand. We lived in worlds we could not inhabit. But we dreamed together. Me in the *piazza* with him and his friends, stirring tiny whirlpools into gold-frothed espressos. Him walking the ancient streets of Oxford where the buildings and our reflections were caught in pools of water on the cobbled stones.

I wished I could cross seas and boundaries and time to be there with him in that room where I always saw his face. We were moths beating themselves against glass trying to find the light, trying to break through the screen, trying to reach that flame that seemed to burn so bright. Love and desire unfolded down bandwidths. Our passion flashing in pixels, reliving and tumbling, sending my mind into a place that did not exist yet, a place that could evolve and change.

It was there in the absence of time, space and light where the story was formed and unfolded like cables of DNA twined with RAM. In those recesses anyone, anything was possible. My bedroom, with its internet connection, became a world of possibility. It was freedom for a night, freedom from the past, it was freedom from me. We created the narrative; we created our world every night where we could transform into who we wanted to be. Yet, every night I bid him sweet dreams, *sogni d'oro*, and logged out of MSN. Logged out of the life I didn't think I could ever have. One that was simply a dream on a screen.

There was no one on my rural estate to teach me about a gay scene, no one I could confide in about my sexuality without it spreading like wildfire across the fields for people to find out. There was no one I knew who was out or I could connect to that was like me. Urbanity can provide the luxury of anonymity, but I was too young, too skint, to venture to London or other cities to explore the scene. Besides, I was too scared to admit to myself that I was gay, let alone confront the reality of having sex with another man. The idea of being gay was so far-flung from my own reality, an image so far from my own truth. You learn to bottle it, seal it and throw it out to sea and hope that it'll be opened in some other time, some other place.

The estate forced me to become a being that could only exist in the depths of the mind. Just like the fairy tales of my childhood, I learned to split myself. While some question the power of words and vocalising something, somehow there isn't validation, a physicality to who you truly are without it. The hardest thing is to not see yourself reflected elsewhere. I lived in purgatory where I waited to know my destination. In public, it was easier to accept being religious and straight. It was easier to accept the narrative I'd been given. Nothing was easy about being queer.

I trawled chat rooms, forums and websites to figure out more about myself and why I was feeling this way. A plug-it-in webcam propped on top of the monitor, pixelated photos and odd usernames, and pages that felt like hours to load – but it was a thrill of connecting and finding out answers in a way that wasn't possible before in our emerging digital world whirred by dial-up sounds. I sought out whether something had gone wrong when I was born, if there were others out there. I was entirely isolated, reflecting a world that didn't reflect my inside. The being I suppressed and had been taught to be ashamed of was breaking the seal. It had needs, it sought validation, it wanted to breathe. I tried to stop but something had tethered me, hooked me up like an ethernet cable, an umbilical cord that wouldn't be cut.

It was a click, that's all it took to overcome my internal firewall to switch to a gay chat room. I traded the labyrinthine estate alleys for the labyrinth of chat rooms. I'd spent my whole life learning how to navigate the world and my public identity, I now had to learn how to navigate this gay new world. How do you step out of that old story and into the new one? I'd already been trying to walk and run in a life that wasn't mine. Now, after starting to admit who I truly was, I had to sprint into fully fledged queerness, with the keyboard and screen as my way in. What happens when, and if, we let out that starved and neglected part that hasn't seen light or love or attention? We are supposed to embody and grapple with this new being, step into a skin that doesn't quite fit, a digital Frankenstein's monster that hasn't been taught language or love or affection. How do we reconcile and love the person experienced and lived on a screen with the physical person that has to pretend to be something else?

We learn language through mimicry: adopting patterns, accents, words from those around us as we develop. From a young age, I was forced to mimic the structures of heterosexual culture as that was all I had been exposed to. For survival, for shame. We adopt what we see: the swag, the cues, the language, the movements. We had parents, family, siblings, friends and others to teach us how to behave. The body, sexuality has a language. I had to learn and navigate my new, hidden identity in isolation. *ASL? Are you top? Bottom? Pos/Neg?* I didn't know what they meant, let alone what I liked. There was no standard or precedent to hold myself up against. These were words and actions beyond my reality and comprehension. I never expected to inhabit this space or live it out.

Yet, despite, or maybe because of, the new, strange language, I found comfort in the snippets of conversations, the people who accepted who they were, or didn't, who were living and experiencing their gayness. It proved that what I had been taught and conditioned to be ashamed of was wrong. We were all the same. We spoke about books, movies, life, weekend plans.

Just like I did with people who were heterosexual. This helped me, but it didn't pull down the walls that had been built around me. It wouldn't help me navigate the prejudices and intolerance around me. I never asked about coming out, how they approached it, what it was like for people to know, because I didn't feel this could happen.

Those chat rooms provided me a virtual world that gave me anonymity, freedom and safety, whereas in the real world I was terrified to be my true self. I stepped into the wonders and terrors of forging a new identity with no restrictions or paradigms. I had to keep my true self in the shadows and those chat rooms gave me the space to find others, allowed me to live my true self in 2D. Just like in real life, I created a persona.

I was able to metamorphosise, transcend borders, possibilities and country lines. I chose who I was and not the person I'd been forced to be. Just for a day, just for a night. There was no past, there was no present. Erase the history and start again. Everything was possible even if just in my mind. For hours a week, I lived beyond the fields and the woods outside my window. I escaped the hate, the stigma, the expectations that lurked down the alleys I grew up on, the corridors I walked down.

I began chatting to a guy in Italy. For weeks he had just been a screen name, a faceless figure somewhere hundreds of miles away. When he suggested we put on our cameras, he was something tangible, even if the footage was pixelated and glitchy. Golden hair, eyes like autumn leaves. I lowered my cam to only show half of my face to protect my identity. In case he didn't think I was attractive. In case somehow someone at home would find out. He had a boyfriend and lived in Italy so it shouldn't have mattered what he thought of me, but deep down I was scared of being rejected after starting to accept who I was.

We chatted most nights, fragmented images of ourselves on the screen, fragments of ourselves. He spoke to me about his performances and sculptures he made at school, taught me about Italian history, art history, psychology, literature. He recommended I read Jeanette Winterson, his favourite author. I looked her up – probably using Ask Jeeves – and read about her work and that she's lesbian. *Oranges Are Not the Only Fruit* was the first book I ever ordered online in case the cashier put two and two together if I'd bought it in a real bookshop. As if by holding it, a red 'G' would sear itself on my skin, for all of the other customers to see. Night after night our own fruit was growing, we were grafting our worlds together to create something new. Through him I escaped from it all, escaped to somewhere else.

After months of chatting, his routines and life became written on my skin: what time he finished school, when his rehearsals would finish, what time he'd have dinner. I'd run from the bus stop at the main road down the hill to my house to get online for when he'd be signing on. There was a pining for him when he wasn't online or when he was out on the weekends or the Tuesdays when I was at lacrosse practice all evening so we couldn't catch up. I smiled when his screenname popped up and the immediate, '*Ciao cucciolo!*' (Hi puppy!). I longed to know what he had been reading, where he had been exploring.

Somewhere lost in translation, in pixels, I fell for him. A feeling I'd never had before with the girls I had dated briefly or drunkenly made out with. The connection was more than just what transmitted between our computers. I thought about him before bed, at school, in the bath. He was an echo in my dreams. He didn't know my past. He didn't see me as different or weird or an anomaly. I didn't have to pretend with him, to be someone I wasn't. I could talk about my love of books and writing and art without fear of being called gay.

I felt stupid for forming an attachment to someone I had never met beyond a screen. Despite our connection, our realities beyond the virtual were opposites: we were two worlds apart and not just geographically. I was on a glass-spattered estate, scared to come out. He was in a sprawling arcaded metropolis where kings of Italy walked. He had had boyfriends; his friends knew he was gay. The borders of my identity were still unfound and limited, the reality I desired caged in the confines of my mind.

Chat rooms gave me a lifeline. I often wonder who and what would have happened if they never came to exist or if I hadn't taken the chance to try them. Would I have truly accepted who I was, taken the leap to meet someone, a guy, or embraced my sexuality without them? Living in the countryside with no representation in the media or books readily available to me, would I have been too scared to admit who I was? It would have been easier to pretend not to do so, to continue the narrative I saw around me. I was forced to live in isolation and secrecy for so long, the impact of this still resonates today, but could have been so much worse if I hadn't felt compelled to seek out the truth and others like me.

Even now, I feel guilty and ashamed about how I first began to understand my sexuality. Yet, it allowed me to live and learn, albeit digitally, when I was so far away from my own community and without any form of education or acknowledgement that being gay was okay. But looking back, and for so many in a similar situation, what else could I have done? I was forced to find these ways to understand what I was feeling when the world wasn't telling me. There was no other option. Would I have run into even bigger risks, leaping into the scene without testing the waters and starting to understand who I was?

Set up the code. Let's automate love. Let's mechanise lust. Download an app, and another one. Let the algorithms choose, it's your choice, always more choice. It's suspended reality, virtual reality, cyberspace. It's preordained, love at first swipe. You, they, can be anyone for a night. Anything is possible, just set up the profile, press start, let's go, let's play a game.

Finding love for life, for a night, on a phone is so commonplace now. Digital advances have allowed us to find people all over the world, it's become the natural way to meet people. It's 2D love in a 3D world. Apps first made their way onto our screens around 2008 and have become a mainstay in our lives. But, queer social networks didn't start with the internet. For centuries, the queer community has been forced to find each other and socialise in creative ways, often ahead of the heterosexual world, because of discrimination, fear and criminalisation.

From as early as Roman Britain there have been varying laws that have either made homosexuality, or 'homosexual acts' such as anal and oral sex, illegal. Ancient civilisations like Rome and Greece accepted homosexuality on various levels depending on class, social and sexual position and job. In Ancient Rome, the most acceptable version of homosexuality was a freeborn man as the active participant in sex, which was deemed more masculine. A lower-class man was viewed as passive and feminine – it was this person who could be prosecuted.[1]

The real anti-gay laws were introduced in Europe as Church and State sought to consolidate power. Abrahamic religions root themselves in natural law where the sole purpose of sex is to procreate, thus legitimising heterosexuality. Homosexual sex defies 'God's order' as it does not beget children. As perceptions of homosexuality grew increasingly negative, laws such as The Buggery Act 1533 introduced the death penalty for sodomy; although no longer carrying the death penalty, homosexuality was not decriminalised in England and Wales until 1967. Modern laws included Section 28 – very much introduced in living memory, in 1988 – which restricted the teaching and promotion of queer issues, as well as laws that curbed same-gender public displays of affection to 'safeguard' the public from 'corruption'. Each of these laws made the possibility of death, incarceration and abuse a stark reality for everyday queer people and famous ones too, like Oscar Wilde and Alan Turing. It forced queer people to live in the shadows, often without knowing if there were others like them or if they were normal. As a result, a range of incredible subcultures formed so queer people could interact and live out their lives and fantasies beyond heterosexual mainstream spaces.

In the eighteenth and nineteenth century, 'molly houses' – a private room in an alehouse, small coffee houses or even entire taverns – allowed gay men to meet each other in secret to socialise or even to have sex. 'Moll' and 'molly' were words used for either a lower-class woman or an effeminate or gay man. The word originates from the Latin, *mollis,* meaning soft or weak: another example of how gay men have been viewed as 'lesser'. The houses wouldn't be unlike today's sticky-floored queer bars with drinking, music and drag competitions. Rictor Norton claims that these subcultures were predominantly created and attended by the 'respectable' working class.[2] Just like in recent history, there were spies, raids, blackmailers and infiltrators who would work to capture, entrap and close down queer venues and activities.

Around this time there grew a community of cruising sites in London, from 'Sodomites' Walk' in Moorfields to the toilets in Temple where there was the first recorded glory hole in 1707. Just like in the twentieth century, a series of codes, signals and phrases were used to signal an interest in love or lust down shadowed alleys. With stringent laws against homosexuality, it forced the community to create a culture and space where they could socialise and find sex in relative safety.

The death penalty for homosexuality was repealed in 1861. Even with the threat of death removed, homosexuals could still face imprisonment, hard labour or sterilisation, on top of the everyday hate, discrimination and prejudice. Homosexuality remained illegal until 1967, whereby it was only partially decriminalised – you could be queer as long as it wasn't in public. Under these dangerous and pressurised conditions, queer people were forced to keep living clandestinely and find spaces to reach out to each other, find love, find sex, to not be alone.

Saunas, or bath houses, have been a longstanding and popular space for gay men to meet. Gay sex in saunas is believed to have been first recorded in Florence during the 1400s. It was considered so salacious that a force, Office of the Night, was created to police sodomy. Saunas have played an integral role throughout gay history to provide safety and anonymity.

Saunas in steamy darkness provided many gay, and curious, men the opportunity to socialise and have sex without the fear of being recognised or caught in a more public setting. They were often deemed safer than other public venues that gay men were forced to use such as cinemas, toilets and open spaces. Their popularity increased in the mid-twentieth century when more and more dedicated gay saunas opened. They weren't solely used for sex but provided a culture where people could drink, socialise and enjoy entertainment away from the traditional bars or fetish parties. They were places to find a 'chosen family' when so many had been rejected by their biological one. After decriminalisation, the AIDS epidemic in the 1980s, moral policing and the rise of hook-up apps, saunas lost their centrality as a communal meeting point. They've further been demonised with the spread of Covid-19 and monkeypox in the 2020s.

It's not just physical spaces that played an important role in enabling gay people to find each other. Body language, codes, signals and even languages were invented to allow gay people to communicate in safety. Sustained eye contact, mimicking actions through to knocks on cubicle doors or foot tapping in particular rhythmic patterns were common acts to signal that you were gay. Physical objects were utilised, such as coloured handkerchiefs positioned in different pockets denoting if you were active, passive or had a fetish. These codes were developed to ensure anonymity from the untrained heterosexual eye so they could avoid harassment, arrest or abuse. A language, Polari, which drew from other marginalised groups, was adopted to communicate in privacy and to form a secret culture.

The provenance of Polari can be traced back several hundred years. It finds its origins in a mix of Italian, Romany and rhyming slang, which over the years was adopted by various outlier groups, including performers, prostitutes, criminals, travellers and sailors. Just like the gay community, all these peoples were stigmatised and abused in different ways, considered to be deviants and on the fringes of society. The gay community proliferated it in the 1950s and '60s to openly converse in public.

Polari wasn't just used for cruising or signalling that you were gay. It was a vital way of constructing identity, giving names to things in the gay world that weren't recognised or known in the hetero mainstream, such as *omee-palone* for a gay man, *palone-omee* for a lesbian. It created a collective identity that allowed gay people to construct their own reality based on their own world and not the one around them. It provided the freedom and safety to embody a community and society that reflected them and not the one imposed on them. Paul Baker discusses how the variants of Polari spoken across London also indicated whether you were working class – by using the East End Polari dialect – or middle–upper class – by speaking the West End version of Polari.[3] It provided privacy and protection, it provided a shared language, it provided freedom, it provided a community when this wasn't possible. After the decriminalisation of homosexuality, its use waned and was no longer needed as the danger, legally at least, to gay people decreased.

Love and lust often had an expiry date in these spaces. Fast love. Gay people were forced to make quick, physical-based decisions about someone, which catalysed the production-line, hypersexualised way many gay men interact to this day. After hundreds of years of some forms of connecting meaning fleeting moments under pressurised conditions, this has translated into apps and online dating. We make instant decisions on an image, and not the person, just like our ancestors had to in public or a sauna. Has this way of meeting people, based on physicality, conditioned us to believe that a relationship can't be sustained and we only deserve brief moments of love and lust?

Gaydar was founded in 1999, Grindr less than 10 years later in 2008. The first time heterosexual friends mentioned a dating app wasn't until 2014 when Tinder's popularity hit dizzying heights. Even at that point, meeting someone from an app was considered dangerous or strange to some heterosexual people. They found the concept bizarre, or worried what people would think of them for finding a partner or a hook-up via a phone rather than in more traditional ways. For gay people, online dating was second nature. Many of us had found ourselves amongst bandwidths, chat rooms and data since the turn of the millennium. This way of dating and meeting people has become integrated into society and is now the standard rather than the exception. Gay people had been doing it for years before, out of necessity rather than novelty.

The Office for National Statistics estimates 2.7 per cent of people aged 16 and over in the UK identify as LGB,[4] and 1 per cent as transgender and non-binary.[5] We are a small proportion of the population, making it harder to meet other queer people especially outside of densely populated cities, highlighting how important queer spaces or apps are in connecting with others. Not just to hook-up or date but to find a community where you are accepted and belong. With homosexuality having been illegal for so long, it shows how invaluable the incredible spaces and subcultures were to our ancestors. It shows the lengths and extent they were forced to go to live out who they were and rid themselves of the isolation they felt in a hostile, heterosexual world. They laid the foundations for the modern gay scene and opportunities that we have today.

We are now in a position of privilege whereby the gay community can move towards the homonormative and we are not faced with the same levels of state-sponsored violence and discrimination. In the UK, at least, we are legal, allowed to marry, have children and socialise without being incarcerated. The move toward homonormativity itself can be viewed as problematic. It brings a dichotomy between 'right' and 'wrong' queerness. One that assimilates heterosexual structures and ideals and imposes them within queer culture; a life whereby we can integrate and pass in heterosexual society. The replication of heterosexual norms within queer identity once again assumes that we should behave, interact and live our lives as if we are heterosexual. It is seen by some as the pinnacle of social integration, the 'better' way. We need to understand the impact of this and how the erosion of queer culture and identity can ostracise those of us who reject having to once again embody heterosexual values.

But has homonormativity, and the shift towards digital, eradicated gay subculture? With the use of hook-up apps like Grindr, cruising and cottaging have been replaced with jumping off the Tube or bus, or simply slipping out of the house or parties or work when someone messages you. More and more gay venues are facing closure, with a 62 per cent decrease between 2006 and 2017.[6] Nights dedicated to fetishes that were so popular in the twentieth century are next to nothing as we have come out of the closet and into the mainstream. Polari's use is basically extinct, a language relegated to a forgotten time, while we bask in our new apparent freedoms. The gay culture created in a pressurised and dangerous situation is something we should feel proud of, a remarkable feat in adversity, rather than feeling the need to sanitise it to reflect heterosexual culture. The culture that was so hard fought for is being pushed to the fringes, swept back into the closet.

As queer people who have been forced to live on the fringes and in shadows, we have been pushed to invent and find spaces where we can speak, thrive, live and love in order to assimilate to the culture, feel accepted and find a space where queer people are not marginalised and can express their identities. Society and law forced us to learn to adapt, hide and transform in a world that despises us, casts us into shadowed lairs and underground spaces. Yet every time we have metamorphosised them into spaces full of magic and laughter and opportunity. In the face of rising hate crime and anti-queer legislation around the world, do we now more than ever need to protect and increase our safe spaces?

Speaking to guys online gave me access to a possibility that couldn't happen in reality. At first it was just a game. In the cables, in the code, wrapped in the HTML and CSS, there were people out there, even if they were faceless and nameless, who were interested in who I truly was. For once in my life, I was able to live out the fantasies that couldn't exist outside of the recesses of my mind in those tiny two-dimensional boxes on a flickering screen. It awakened a dormant feeling, a tied-up person who had been locked away deep inside. Online was where I had my gay birth.

Entering those chat rooms, in my head I convinced myself if I kept a persona, it was fine, it wasn't gay. Fear forces us to become liars or hide. I lied to myself out of fear. The very thought of being gay terrified me. I had been taught by Catholicism how homosexuality was an aberration of nature. The years of bullying on the estate had conditioned me to believe that being gay was wrong, the years of no queer representation and education at school, the very thought of what I could be wasn't acceptable. By pretending to be someone else online, it created a shield as I wasn't living it out in reality. It was all a game of make-believe, shapeshifting. My whole life, I had been fictionalising who I was, except this time around it was done through data.

Inhabiting an interior life without anyone to confide in and trying to mimic the heterosexual world around me taught me to carry my burdens, problems and issues alone. Living a lie in my bedroom did untold damage on my mental health from carrying that secret. I kept it all bottled up as I didn't have anyone to share it with. Entering the gay world, which is basically beginning an entirely new life, after living for so long in a perceived state of heterosexuality, comes with its risks. Harbouring so much shame and insecurity and self-hate for myself without adequate education fostered the conditions for me to be taken advantage of later. Living in a vacuum with no proper queer support, education and representation has meant some of us seeking validation in the unlikeliest and unhealthiest of ways. What type of love for ourselves do we develop when we have been taught, forced, to live as secrets?

Whether through physical or virtual spaces or by creating new languages, we have evolved to overcome the discrimination and hate. We found ways to reach out to each other in order not to be alone. Many of these spaces, from the molly houses to the ballroom scene in America, have been driven by working-class, Latinx, Black and trans people who have been forced to flee their homes to make new ones, who have lived in unaccepting and unforgiving places, who have needed people just like them. We have had to invent and find ways to communicate, reach out, socialise and love in ways the heterosexual world hasn't. We continue to revolutionise and evolve. Chat rooms allowed me to have my own evolution.

After a year of chatting, the Italian man asked me to visit in the summer of 2008. I looked at hotels that were too expensive for me to stay in on my part-time job's wage. *Stay with me*, he said. Stay with you, lay with you, be with you, was all I could think about. It was an opportunity to learn Italian, visit the cities I could live in if I got the grades to go to university, to finally meet him.

Without hesitation, I booked flights with Ryanair, 15 July 2008, not long after turning 18. I didn't stop to check myself and think about who and what may be waiting for me on the other side of the arrivals gate. At 17, wrapped up in my insecurities, naivety and excitement, all I could think about was the prospect of discovering a world where I could belong, to finally live out who I was. I had been looking for a prince since childhood, I just didn't realise what power someone could wield over you once you placed a crown on their head. I didn't remember that every fairy tale has its sinister side, two sides to every coin, behind glamour, what could be hiding.

I found myself in chat rooms, found love on a pixelated cam, and continued to blur the lines between my fact and fictional self. I'd reached the point where I no longer knew if I were fact or fiction. It had its own force, a narrative with a life of its own with an ending I no longer knew I wanted. Little did I know that when I pressed the button to buy those cheap tickets to Italy, full of anticipation and excitement, my whole life would change. A beginning that would birth a new me. A narrative with a life of its own was beginning that I couldn't stop. A beginning that I thought would be my happily ever after.

Chapter Seven

Watery pathways filled with red and blue and pink and white light, like lost dreams and wishes, guided us through the city. We weaved through tiny streets where sheets swayed above in the night like ghostly brides, our reflections in the water like the drowned souls of gondoliers trapped forever in its surface. Masked figures with empty sockets lurked at corners dealing in love, lust, chances. Will you take the chance? No time to consider, no time to second guess. Love and the night don't wait, they jump from the lips and slip off into the sighs of the water. Empty masks dangled from ribbons, yet to be bought, yet to be assumed. Pay your price, who will you become? Freedom from you just for a moment, just for the night. Who will you become? You decide.

I hadn't realised that a trip to Venice was part of the plan. I was swept up from the airport and bundled into a carriage. Who says that love sweeping you off your feet is only figurative? In a city of disguises with narrow streets that glinted, where shadows lurked, was there a better city to have found and lost myself in, given where I'd grown up, hiding in the alleys of the estate?

We were strangers in the dark, jumping on ferry boats, skipping the fares. Not knowing where we'd end up, taking our chances. Roll the dice, the odds are in your favour. We passed under the Bridge of Sighs, the last place prisoners saw before the bars closed behind them, not knowing the price we'd pay. His hand brushed mine. The green-brown eyes holding mine a little longer than normal. Stolen glances, thoughts unspoken then forgotten. Sighs dropping in the waters cascading as I felt my heart, all the rivers in me, begin to flow towards him, ready to be imprisoned by that stranger called love. We were there just for the night. A night is long enough for possibilities to be fulfilled, for hidden secrets to be revealed. As the night deepened, we found ourselves deeper in that labyrinth city. We unwound thread behind us to find our way back but we'd never find the end again.

We asked an elderly woman in a doorway for directions. Down back streets and across bridges where gondolas ferried faceless people, lost souls to unknown destinations in the shadows. They carried coins with them for payment. We followed her instructions to the word, her whispers of where to go and which alleys would take us back to the hostel. We stood staring at a brick wall, the dead end the woman had directed us to. We saw her later that night and she smiled at us and disappeared into the night, into the water. She gave directions, doesn't mean they'll get you the ending you want. That's life.

We sat together on a jetty, a wine bottle placed between us, our legs dangling over the edge as stars thrashed in the lagoon's currents. His friend had gone to shower before bed, it was the first time we'd been alone since I had arrived the day before. As I ate, the waves lapping against the petrified wood, I stole glances of him as he talked looking out to the horizon. Our fingers grazed as we both reached for the bottle at the same time.

'Do you think you'll sleep with a man?' He asked, his eyes filled with the shifting dark lagoon. Wine lets the tongue flow and secrets unravel. He stared, waiting for me to reply. I waited for him to kiss me. Take the chance, take the opportunity.

'I don't think so,' I replied, swigging the wine from the neck. Chance passed. He squeezed my hand and looked at me through his fringe and smiled. The flash of a gap between his two front teeth. The thump of my heart. The flush of my skin from his touch. I was a stranger to love. I didn't need to buy one of the masks the vendors flogged on the street. My heart had always worn a mask hidden in the caverns of my chest. I danced alone in my own masked ball, spinning in mirrored rooms. I wasn't prepared for a stranger to be the one to pull it away and lead me in a different type of dance.

In the hostel room it was so hot that I slept in my underwear. If I could have taken them off, and my skin too, I would have done it in an instant. Mosquitoes whined in that tiny room and drank deeply from me. I tossed and rolled in the thickness of the dark, clammy air, they glanced over at me as they whispered and giggled to each other. He was just feet away, yet so far. Outside the window, where the oily lagoon lay, Venice moved with the currents, never still, as love and hopes gasped and drowned in the black canals.

I've always loved taking trains. They're the quickest route out, to leave one place and stumble into another. In those carriages, people and scenery shift and change constantly. Nothing stays the same for long. Little boxes full of strangers together, all heading in the same direction, but all with different destinations. Some get off, some get on, some stay until the very end. A silent woman with ivory hair and her hat pulled down over her eyes, the man at her elbow who pulled out an orange rose from a bouquet and handed it to me without a word. My guide, who, despite all the hours on a webcam, I had really only known for a few days in 3D. He was asleep, head resting against the window, his friend drawing in biro in her notebook.

I gazed out the window, my reflection staring back at me, at the shifting landscape, towns rushing by in a second, lakes stretching out to the horizon. I wasn't sure who it was that stared back at me. Currents had altered, something inside me was moving. I started to cry. Error detected; something was broken. The confusion, the longing, the weight of what I wanted but didn't know if I could ever have it or how to do it. The emotion that had never been felt before, the guilt intrinsically tied to it. The unknowing about who and what I was, and what this meant as I looked at him, his legs stretched out between mine.

His friend smiled at me and held my hand. She turned it over and wrote on my palm with her pen, closed my fingers up over it and went back to drawing, without a word said between us. I uncurled my fingers and in capital letters she'd written, *It's just a moment it will pass.* It's a phrase that I've kept with me ever since she imprinted it on my skin. This moment will pass, he will pass, what I felt will pass. Everything is a moment: love, night, emotion, sadness. They're all temporary. Nothing is ever ours to keep forever. Not that I could believe it then.

We all went to shower, change and rest before heading out to dinner. Another friend waited for us outside the restaurant. Hair dip-dyed red, red skirt, red shellac nails that held a glowing cherry-flavoured cigarette languidly between shiny red lips. She kissed me on both cheeks, something I was still trying to get used to. Left cheek then right cheek, always two times. I'd already embarrassed myself by breaking the rules. She had an American twang and I asked if she was from, or had lived, in the States.

'I've just watched too much *Sex and the City*, darling,' she replied as she flicked the cigarette butt away and swept into the restaurant. I knew from that moment I'd love her. We shared bowls of bread dipped in balsamic and olive oil, coiled ammonite pastries, platters of cured meats, gnocchi sticky with cheese and cracked pepper. Over wine I listened to them debate philosophers and books, communist politics and the inadequacies of state education. They seemed so much more clued up than me, so much better read. They admired the men and women who walked past our table in English so the objects of their attention wouldn't understand. I'd never sat at a table before hearing these types of arguments, where being queer was so natural. I drank it all in as deeply as I had drunk the wine. I couldn't have felt more at home, somewhere that was so far from home.

On the drive back, he and I carried on the debates. Comparing Italian and British politics, education, culture, manners. He nicknamed me the 'Victorian boy' for my posture and prudishness when talking about sex. He punched me in the arm when he disagreed, as if we were best friends or brothers. When we got back, we sat across from each other at the red Formica dining table. The room was stencilled with vine leaves and grapes. We were finally only divided by a table instead of sea, borders and impossibility but still, for a moment, it seemed like we didn't know what to do, what to make of each other.

'Goodnight, Mike.' He stood up and closed the other bedroom door behind him. We went to bed in separate rooms with barely any words passed between us. I tossed in his bed, under half-empty sheets, in the heavy heat. Thinking of him just metres away behind a wall, no longer behind a computer. Wondering why he didn't share the bed with me, if I wasn't good looking enough, interesting enough, in good enough shape for him. There were cries of words I'd not yet learned out from the windows and courtyards, the cranking of a city at night and the bars of light pushing through the shutter slats. So different to the sway of the woods, like soft waves breaking, the cry of the owl, that I listened to in my own bed at home.

We spent the day exploring, being steered around the city with his hand on the small of my back. Down arcades built to protect the King of Italy from the rain as he took his walks down to the river. We walked across *piazze* where he pointed out Masonic sculptures and hidden demonic figures. In churches he showed me optical illusions where devils looked down at you from the roof. I snuck glances at him when he was looking up or pointing out something, drawn to the jut of his jaw, noticing how his eyes changed between green and brown as clouds passed the sun. He told me how this city was the point where the good and evil triangles of the world met, where people sacrificed animals and left trails of blood in the catacombs to find their way back home. I spent the day wondering whether that triangle was inside me: gay, working-class, Catholic. My own unholy trinity.

His collared shirt and tailored trousers showed off the 'V' shape of his body, while I stood next to him in my oversized jeans and flip-flops. He recounted the history, the eras, the magic as we went from palace to tomb to piazza, showing me the bullet holes in buildings from when Napoleon rode through the city with his sword slicing the sky. A statue holding up a cup out to the Alps that was supposed to show the direction of the Holy Grail. I wondered if I had found mine and what would happen if I drunk from that goblet.

That night, he knocked on the door and asked if he could stay with me. I nodded that it was fine. He lit the blue candles in an open old suitcase next to the bed, leaving them melting into the lining as he turned off the lights. He lifted the sheets and slotted himself next to me just in his underwear. I could feel the heat of his body, the smell of his bergamot and wood perfume, the mint on his breath. He turned, eyes shut, and his fringe fell across his brow. Lips pressed as if he were waiting for a kiss. The liminal space just a handspan; a handspan from holding each other. I couldn't.

The windows were left open and the shutters pulled down. The night was hot and sticky. The bumps of his spine stuck out in between the lines of muscle that divided his back in two like a pearl necklace pulled tight. That first night we both slept in our underwear, the sheets off, I lay awake, aware of the proximity of his body, the heat from his flesh, the dense night, the slits of streetlight through the shutter slats, the tautness of his muscle, the hardness of him against me as he eventually pulled me in.

He opened his eyes and took his time looking at me, flicking over my face, into my eyes, the medical alert amulet on my bare chest, back to my eyes. He held them there. Mouth slightly parted as if ready to say something. Something painful, something frightening. He said nothing at all. As he held me, I became aware of everything around me in the thickening silence – the shouts out in the courtyard, the neighbour sneezing. It made us laugh into each other, breaking the trance.

It had been four days that I had waited for this, following him down canals and across regions in carriages. I'd waited a whole year before that. Every moment I measured the distance between us. The year we spent hundreds of miles separated but connected by dial-up routers and pixelated webcams. The hand span as we drank coffee opposite each other. The centimetres between our legs on the train back from Venice. The arm-length on this bed where the white sheets seemed interminable, blending into the white curve of his back. I measured the times I could have breached those distances and slid my hand over his, reached across and stitched our bodies together.

We lay on the bed, sheets half falling over the edge, bodies entangled with the lacy night around us. Trying not to tremble as his arms tightened around my ribs. The bed soaked in shadow and expectancy. Disentangle, retangle. Repeat.

My pulse grew, through my bones, out through my fingers and across his skin. Unsure of how I should be, what I should do in this moment, with a man. To pull away, to give in, to let the graze of his lips against mine become something more.

'Can I kiss you?' he whispered looking me in my eyes. He asked permission as if he could feel the conflict in me. He pressed his lips against mine. I didn't pull away.

'Was it okay? Did it feel different?'

'It felt normal. Like I was home.'

He smiled, flashing the gap between his two front teeth. Kissed me again. It was unlike any kiss I'd had before. A whole new language in my mouth.

'We don't have to do anything else if you don't want to.' I told him I wasn't ready yet. He held me tight as if he wanted to be under my skin, coiling my hair around his finger. I fell asleep in his arms.

The next day was another blur of streets and sights. In the evening, we watched the sunset over the river, the oranges and reds and pinks, weaving its way through the city. He reclined back, the wind ruffling his hair as he shielded his eyes with his right hand and a cigarette in the other blowing smoke out to the sky as if to look for portents. The river rushed beside us. Time rushed around us while we thought we had all the time in the world. We shared aperitivi under the hanging lamps in the arcades, shadows dancing around us, as our eyes danced over each other.

There was a hunger, last night was another aperitivo that had started a craving and it wasn't going to be satiated by the snacks in front of us. He sipped at a mojito, and I thought of my lips sugar crusted from kissing them after, and watched the piazza fill up with teenagers and lovers meeting up for the evening. Old couples gathered around tables sipping espresso in tiny cups, stirring spoons, stirring yarns while we headed back home.

When he locked the door shut, he pushed me against the wall and kissed me. We stripped ourselves as though we were unravelling bandages to reveal something new and tender. With each bandage taken off, he peeled away the hate, the guilt, the fear until all that was left was passion. I traced my tongue along the spirals of his ear like a conch where I heard drowning men. He tasted of lime and sugar and I wondered what my own kiss tasted like.

He took my hand, pressed it against his and closed our fingers together. Strangely, this act seemed the most intimate. We forget what our hands touch. The cold metal from a watch in the morning, the cotton between fingertips as a shirt is dropped to the floor, the stickiness of resin on palms, an earlobe cold from the wind, the small of the back when being pulled into an embrace. When does touching become feeling? What is it that makes the neurons remember, that makes the brain, the heart register that something is more than just a touch? My toes clung to his ankle, his fingers crept around my heart as if we were both scared the other would slip from the embrace and escape out the window, as if this had never happened. It's underneath the sheets where we create fictions of ourselves.

I sent myself through my fictions, through all the other bodies I'd had to live: the boy in pink boots swinging from a bough of a tree, the kid sprinting through the alleys to get home before the other kids got him, the man who lay next to a woman with the bed like a canyon between them. All the different people I had had to be until I reached this point, where he held me, the real me. Was this the point, where the lines between my fact and fiction self no longer existed? In the city at the centre of good and evil, I was finally allowed to align the parts of my identity. Neither was good, neither was evil as I'd been taught. Just a central point of light called me. Under different skies, far from home, my past didn't matter, who I was didn't matter. I could define who I was.

He twined my necklace around his index finger, so the pendants dangled between us. St Michael on one side, protector, defender, destroyer of sin. Little did I know that he wouldn't protect me from *that* sin, nor would he protect me from the men who conquered my heart. The other an SOS talisman to alert doctors to my medical condition. One to protect me physically, the other to protect me spiritually. Failing to do both.

I used my finger to draw circles and spirals across his body down to the point where pale skin and shadow played with each other. He whispered that he wished he could be under my skin to feel what I was feeling. All he needed to do was to look in my eyes. I clung tightly to his heel with my toes, and in that embrace I unknowingly had found my own Achilles heel. His eyes dropped, like moon slits, his arm resting over me. I had no coins to keep them shut. No coins for the journey, for the next story.

We visited palaces and hunting lodges, had sex in their landscaped gardens next to grottos and lakes. We lay naked in the mountains next to a basin of water filled by a waterfall, surrounded by trees and flowers in bloom where cicadas sang like land-wrecked sirens. It was the cup of the world and the world was ours, together. The trees' branches above us, an open rib cage, my heart in the centre ready to be plucked out. The heat shimmering off the rocks, his finger running across the surface of the water, my lips leaving invisible kisses on his skin.

He took me on a tour in the Egyptian Museum to admire artefacts and tombs and sarcophagi. Whispering secrets and spells in my ear. In the glass cases I saw my own sarcophagus staring back at me, the mummified version of me deep inside that I'd wrapped up and sealed in without regret. We trekked up into the mountains to the abbey, the Sacra di San Michele, with that other friend, the woman in red. A priest drove past us, unwound the window and made the sign of the cross. We laughed that he was praying for the two gay guys and the woman in a crop top and miniskirt and how the Abbey would burn as soon as we entered. Looking over the walls, the sky and earth were split in two by rugs of grey cloud, the monastery so high, so close to God that even the mountain peaks seemed like small tacks in the sky.

I'd felt close to God at one point, so close that I'd considered joining the priesthood. I'd walk down the aisle every Sunday, head down, unable to meet His gaze knowing that I had my own struggle pinned to a cross inside. I had to sacrifice for the greater good, to absolve my sins. Sat in the confession box with just a thin screen and a voice whispering back but a well of judgement being passed, the well of sins and fantasies that I could never confess. As the years passed, I knew that who I was and what Catholicism expected of me weren't compatible. At first, I wondered if God had existed and had died as a way to explain the evils and pain in the world, why He had allowed me to go through the pain and hurt. The more I studied science and philosophy and the world, I doubted He existed at all, and I began to analyse the ways that religion has used its status to control and subject and hurt in order to assert one vision of what counts as right.

Now I had finally lived out those sins. They were no longer dreams and fantasies but the stigmata on my body, the wounds of love and desire. His body and his words and his image healed me, and filled me with joy and hope and life. Gay, working class and Catholic. This was a trinity that I still doubted could ever find harmony within me.

There, at the zenith of the world and nature, with the flagstones cold against my bare feet, the incense wavering in the wind, the absolute quietness. I sat on that wooden bench alone listening to the monks and I cried thinking of the child swinging his legs from the pew looking up at his dad, giggling with his brothers. I mourned the loss of my faith and the familiarity and the ease and the comfort it had given me, the narrative that was so easy to follow. I cried for the life I was to lose, the one I couldn't return to after what I had experienced and who I had become. I cried for the life I had known that was never going to be the same. I cried for the life I didn't know how to live or where that narrative would lead me to. I had slashed and burned the ivy and creepers and vines that had grown up around me and kept me in my constructed reality.

The light was blinding without it, burning, searing the back of my eyes. I pushed the balls of my hands into my eyes and doubled over, my head resting on the pew in front, and shook from trying not to cry out loud and disturb the peace. I cried because I was scared, so entirely overwhelmed and terrified of what I was feeling, what I had done, scared for the boy that I had lost. Christ have mercy on me for what I had done, for what was to come, for the life that was to unfold. There was no going back, there could be no penance for what I had done. I had coiled myself around the sin I had been born with, ritualised to believe, and taken a bite from it. The juices sweet and sharp and full in my mouth as they dribbled from my lips.

I left the chapel and he was leaning against the railings. The mountains dropped behind him, and he waved when he saw me in the archway. Taking the bite was worth it. The St Michael that hung around my neck was warm against my chest from the heat of the day. My heart burning for him.

In the mornings, we stretched out in the summer heat. Origami sheets and origami bodies folded into swans, and bodies folded into love. Folded and pressed, and trying to unfold ourselves from the shapes and forms and sculptures we'd been pressed and folded into. He pulled me onto his stomach and we lay there pressed against each other. Breathing, staring into the other's eyes, the stick of our skin together. He looked at me as if he couldn't get enough, wanted to be under my skin, consume me. He kneaded my palm with his finger until it was warm like a worn penny. Locked our hands together and the tingle of his fingers down my back, drawing invisible threads across my back, the web of us. It had been a new sensation for just a few weeks but had felt like a habit formed years before.

In the evenings, we sat at the piano, him behind me with his chin resting on my shoulder and his hands atop mine teaching me how to play. Playing our song, lost in his tune, in the melody we were creating together. We were moon-drenched on top of crisp sheets and crisper skin, backs turned and reflecting each other, clinging to each other tightly under twilight. Never wanting the press of his lips to leave my skin, never wanting to stop hearing 'Buongiorno' or 'Buona notte' with his arms around me, thinking how none of the world mattered. Freedom was our beloved, and it shifted with our dreams, a rowboat to sail across the ocean. Never knowing quite what was forming, how to handle what was happening between us, and what internal storms were coming. Our skin stuck together; bodies curled like one big question mark. The question mark that formed in me every time I looked at him. It was in that room where that question was solved but a new question mark grew bigger.

He a sculptor, me a writer, we both liked to create new characters without knowing who we were ourselves. We were just kids trying to come to terms with and unlock what love and emotion and distance meant. Unpick what we meant, who we were, let alone with someone else in the equation.

Time doesn't wait for anyone, and it was running out. Love doesn't just sweep us off our feet. Love disrupts, it shatters, it breaks boundaries and barriers, it crosses time zones and tears down masks. Love impales. I travelled across countries, down pathways, networks and ethernet cables that crossed over borders and city lines. I flew across countries, earth and seas to find love. When I found it, I found that love had an expiry date.

The last morning, I woke up when time was in suspension. When the darkness was in equilibrium with the light and everything was possible and endless. Just for a second, until the illusion was broken, and the sky brightened, and the room was dripping full of light like honeycomb, a warm, gloopy heat as if it were preserving the moment. The moment where I turned and watched him sleep with his lips pursed, reaching out to find me, it was that moment I realised it was all an illusion. The light shattered it. I had to go home; this couldn't go on forever. I had to return to my reality. Everything is temporary. Everything was possible and impossible. The depression in the bed next to me shifted as he lifted his weight and I felt the pressure of his body against mine as he held me with his eyes closed. As he did every morning, as he would do for one last time.

Love is not an equation, it's not a myth. Love can impale, it can consume. My body was covered in bruises from his lips. While the bruises he left on me faded, the wound he created would linger so much longer. We clung to each other at the airport. He wiped the tears from my face and handed me an envelope with my name, sealed and stamped with red wax on the back for me to open on the plane. We kissed each other on the cheek unable to kiss properly in public.

'Ciao,' he said.

'Ciao,' I whispered back. A word that is both a goodbye and a hello but neither, somewhere in between. As if it never happened at all. We said neither hello nor goodbye, we never even really met. Trapped between words where I could never admit back home that I said 'ciao' with a smile and 'ciao' with tears to someone I loved, and they would never know, could never know. He asked me turn around for one last look because that's the way it should have been. He should have been my Eurydice where I sent him back to the underworld, banished to the caverns of my imagination to haunt me in my sleep.

On the shuttle bus everyone got off to board the plane. I clung to my backpack and couldn't move. The thought of returning home and returning to my old life and skin, hiding who I was once again, not knowing when and if I would see him again froze me. Not knowing when and if I would see the real me again hurt me. I was being ripped from this new world, from his arms, to go back to one I didn't want or belong to. Would I turn to a pillar of salt for returning home? Was that last glance in fact condemning my own Eurydice-self back to the underworld as it couldn't live out in the light and flesh? If I ran back, would I catch him in time, could I stay longer and not go back home? I fell into the orbit of a life that didn't belong to me, pulled down by gravity into a stranger's world, unsure how I'd escape from its force, the pull back to the one where I belonged. It shattered my world, spun it on a new axis. How was I supposed to right something with so much gravitational force? The bus conductor ushered me out. Chance lost.

Once we took off, I opened the red wax seal and unfolded the letter. He spoke about our time together, the memories, the places we'd seen, the things we had done. They played in my head like a reel of film. There in my mind, the laws of physics didn't work: time paused, restarted, rewound. I would relive those moments where in reality it could never exist again. Was there any point in asking for a destination that could never exist?

He said it wasn't a goodbye, but, as they say in Italian, *a presto*, see you soon. I cried reading about our time together. *Memento mori*, everything finishes; everything changes. I clung to the letter as I was shuttled back to the woods that would grow deeper and darker around me, with the mask in my backpack that I'd bought in Venice. Pay your price, who will you become?

When the plane landed in Stansted, the weight of who I was and what I had done overwhelmed me. With the tear tracks still on my face, I deleted his number. I hoped this would erase what had happened in those two weeks. It'd clear me from being gay, any association of the things I had done. Humans aren't computers, we're not data; the shame, the guilt, the love couldn't be wiped as easily. What I lived and experienced couldn't be erased.

Pulling into the estate everything was the same. The guys launching the football into the air, the screams as kids slipped down the slide, my bedroom the same. My life was the same, but I wasn't. I was back in the life I didn't want to return to, had never felt I belonged in. The true me had been suspended in front of me for the briefest of moments. I took the chance, and the prize had an expiry date. It could only ever exist as a moment in time. Just for a night, just for a moment. Now I had to step back into that skin I had lived in for eighteen years, keep pretending that I was heterosexual, masculine, normal. There was no one for me to talk to. I was too scared about coming out and what could happen if it was taken the wrong way. I could only live with the memories of those two weeks inside my head, talk about the worries and the fears and the anxieties to myself. Try to understand what had happened to me, who I was by myself, what to do with all the emotions that I'd experienced for the first time. The woods that had set me free as a kid had never felt more trapping, growing up and around me with no way to find my way back out.

I was terrified that somehow everyone would find out. They would be able to sense some shift in me, the way I moved, where my eyes lingered, how I talked. Understand who I truly was now that the mask had been taken off and I had lived out my desires in a different land. When I arrived in Italy, I had no past. I could be who I wanted to be, create the person who I should be. It was anonymous intimacy. I didn't have that at home; I had a past, a present and a future that was wrapped up in expectations and a narrative I didn't want to be part of. I no longer lived in a prelapsarian world; I'd bitten from the apple and I waited for the fall. What would happen if someone knew, if I told my family or friends who I truly was and what I had done that summer. My terror was no fault of theirs, but what society has constructed for people to believe about queer people, how queer people are made to feel about themselves and what could happen to us and does happen to us.

I know how privileged I am in receiving the support and love from my family for who I am. Not all queer people are as lucky. Porchlight reports that 30 per cent of homeless youth are LGBTQ.[1] LGBTQ+ homelessness charity AKT reports that 24 per cent of young LGBTQ+ people are at risk of homelessness. Half of their respondents (50 per cent) said that they were scared that if they expressed their identity it would lead them to be evicted.[2] So many queer youths live in the constant fear that the ones who should care for us will turf us out for simply being who we are. This fear, as the report finds, is very much a reality. Some are kicked out, some flee abuse, others leave because they're scared of what may happen if they're found out. Despite the representation, despite the improved equality laws, there are still views that being queer is wrong to the extent of forcing a child to live on the street.

I'd hidden myself back in the cage that I had built for years. Watching the branches outside my window, crying, in fear of what I was. Not wanting it to be true. I'd turned into what the kids across the estate had always said I was. I didn't know whether to be relieved that I could finally admit I was, or be disgusted with myself, angry that they had been right. What I'd always feared, resisted. I knew I had to try and understand and accept who I was, away from the estate, where I didn't have to worry. Deep in my cupboard, I hid the letter with the red seal. The words memorised, the imprint of his lips against mine memorised. Destined to become just that, a memory.

In a matter of weeks, a different envelope was waiting for me to open. The one that would change my life.

Chapter Eight

Lights slapped my face as I rested my forehead against the window. Emergency lights, headlights, reversing lights threaded through the night like a neon necklace. A dance floor for the snow-trapped. Snow crystals layered the car windows, glowing pink like bleeding heart petals. In each flake there were millions of reflections of myself gazing back out, trapped and collapsing as they melted from the car's heat.

My eyes filled with pools of red, white, blue from the lights outside. Glazed like the cherries bobbing in a Cherry Coke float. My eyes stung from being up at 2 a.m. to get to Stansted on time. My breath fogged the window, uncovering years of glyphs and doodles we made on the windows as kids. Messages from the past to uncover by the present me. The chain of cars stuck in snow, all trying to get to places, destinations unknown, not moving at all, trapped in a moment.

This was my moment to fly and the snow crept in, the ice spiralled, the night thickened. Months previously, at the zenith of summer, I had held an envelope that would have been my opportunity to move from the estate and potentially explore what I had released that summer. I stood in my school's sports hall. I held the envelope with both hands. Clinging to the paper, clinging to the future. The doors and windows I'd had half open my whole life were about to be flung open. The edge of the woods was within sight, the thicket and the pine becoming sparser as the horizon grew closer. The place where the swifts flew to in their last dance.

I pulled it open and unfolded the paper, biting my lower lip as I scanned the grades. I didn't get the ones I needed. Missed by one, missed by too much. Work hard and it'll pay off, my teachers said. I did all of it and it wasn't good enough. Fairy tales warned not to enter the woods, but I'd already been there my whole life. You're not supposed to find your way out, stay where you belong. I tried to rise above my station and the woods grew up around me. The ivy creeping around my arms, the sap filling my veins, branches growing around my rib cage until my heart was encased inside.

The hours spent revising into the night. The practice exams. The focus. Turning down parties to do extra reading. This shouldn't have happened. I'd worked so hard, put everything I had into making sure I got the grades to go to university. It was my golden ticket to get away. To prove everyone wrong in my childhood, to prove to myself that I was better than what they thought of me, for my parents who had invested so much. There were no tears but confusion, shock, emptiness. I felt exhausted, my body sagging from the deflation. From the four years I had been working towards this moment; for it all to culminate with an envelope hanging limply in my hand.

I'd been riding high that summer, so high that at some point the wax on my wings would melt from the blaze. I fell and crashed. The wax hardened across my skin. I stared up at the sun, shattered and watched the summer weaken, the leaves fall and the bony branches scratch at my bedroom window at night. The woods creeped thicker around me, the shadows growing longer, the night darker. The days spent walking through arcaded streets, the nights curled up with him, seemed all but a dream. The swifts were due to do their last dance of the summer. They'd soon be gone out into the horizon, and into the future, leaving me behind to dance alone. I was staying behind on the estate where I had been told I belonged.

Wrapped up in a jumper and coat, I couldn't have been further removed from what I'd imagined during the summer just past. Under blazing heat and foreign skies, I'd loved and lost, travelled Europe and been on the cusp of going to one of the top universities. That summer had seemed like it would never end, it had been a liminal space. The longing for his body against mine, our bodies grilled on the bed and the love and guilt crusting on my hands, body and lips. Leaving behind the estate, heterosexuality, home to find a new one at university. But instead, the half-open doors were closed shut, the windows locked.

We weren't the type to wallow. Pick yourself up, get on with things, figure out a different plan. Throughout the darkness of that winter, I worked in a stock room with no windows tagging clothes. Find the label, place the base by the hem and push through the pin, an ink tag for clothes over £50, place on a hanger or fold depending on the garment, place on a rail or in a box and send down to the floor. Repeat for eight hours, five days a week for five months.

I didn't get into university so I figured, who needs it? I didn't need a course to move abroad and learn a language, I'd do it myself. I bought a ticket without any language skills and without a return. One ticket to Italy without the fear of having to come back and hide who I was again. I'd build my own Italy without the precursor of us. Like a lighthouse it pulled me back, following that light out of the darkness, away from the rocks and out on the wine-dark ocean where the sirens waited. Lulling, luring, drifting me back to those desires. I followed that column of light, disappearing, reappearing into the night, never sure whether to safety or danger. With the crunch of the snow and ice under the tyres, we slid our way to Stansted. I was on my way back not knowing whether I'd return home.

The colonnades and churches were blanketed with snow, the greys frozen and glinting in the low sun. I stood outside the train station waiting for my friend, the one whose words were ghostly remains on my palm. Snowflakes layering my eyelids as I clung onto my suitcase looking around for her. Slivers of Italian muffled under wind and snow. When she came around the corner she jumped and clung to me. I lifted her up with her legs wrapped around me spinning in the snow. We fell to the ground laughing, my suitcase knocked over. On the floor she held my face between her gloved hands, smiling down at me.

'You came back,' she said.

'I'm here.' There was something both comforting and terrifying about acknowledging that. I'd moved to a city I barely knew with people I barely knew. Hoping I'd somehow make ends meet, meet people, make a life. Everyone else had gone to university so I had to make it work. We dragged my bags through the big entrance where a Virgin Mary painting hung, forever looking out for me, and up the four flights of stairs. The house that had been empty of things but full of dreams the previous July was now fully furnished: a huge painting of a centaur throwing a paper airplane in the living room, guitars, a small table with a shiny plastic red covering and a bed for me.

I leaned against her bedroom door frame as we chatted and stared out to the balcony. There where the three of them had pinned me down and pulled off my shirt as I squirmed and laughed so he could show off my body. Like I – my body – was his. Where he smoked from the balcony out to the night, the lips that I could still feel on my skin, on one of our last nights together. Standing here alone, it was so different to the heat of that summer, the balcony doors now firmly shut, and this was just a memory being projected on the snow-dusted pane. I shook my head and reminded myself that this was my space, my place to define.

It turned out it wasn't as simple as I thought. The city was full of him, of us, the city was defined by those memories. I walked a lot during my time there, hours a day, on arcaded roads, down alleys, through pineapple-adorned palaces, across parks filling with shadow and the crunch of my feet on frost-tipped grass. I knew he'd moved away, but still there'd be the thump of my heart, my chest rising as my breath quickened, my throat tightening when I turned down an alley and there was a cafe or bar we'd been at; or walking through a park or piazza and expecting to turn to see the flash of the gap in his teeth as he laughed and his hair was ruffled by the summer wind.

The memories an imprint on my brain like a film reel, unspooling and projected on the back of my eyes where the spectres of us constantly played out. The spectres of us, a dream of a summer long gone. So, I erased the memories, pushed them down and away like I'd done my whole life. I wanted to forget them and him rather than live with them. I didn't understand at that point that the good and the bad need to coexist in order to grow. The good thing about memory is that it can be re-recorded, rewritten, written over. Days slipped into months, and the splitting headaches I had when trying to decipher Italian had passed. Words that I translated in my head no longer needed translating, and while his presence lurked, I had new friends and memories without him. I found students at the university who I gave private English lessons to in my bedroom. I attended student protests, listened to debates about revolution, injustices, the rights of workers, communism, economic failures and political philosophies. They wanted to change the world; what I had learned and knew about the world was being changed. Each day that passed, my own was changing.

With the friend, whose red highlights had faded back to blonde, we sat under the spring sun in the piazza watching the skater boys, rolling and smoking cherry flavoured handmade cigarettes and slurping our frappes as we admired them. We ate cake, talked about literature and writing in the park, she helped teach me Italian and snuck me into her English Literature university classes. We had parties where guitars were played, faces reflected in the curve of wine glasses, lips stained red, while art, literature and the nature of life were debated over cigarettes flung off the balcony. The slow roar of the flame as the macchinetta gurgled up espresso in the morning, legs resting on the balcony blowing out cigarette smoke to halo the weak spring sun.

My best friend from the UK came to visit and we toured northern Italy, hopping across platforms and into carriages. We dragged a suitcase down cobbled streets, declaring our love to the spring wind on Juliet's balcony, mulling whether to sleep in train stations to save money, eating polpette and spaghetti we had cooked with a 2-litre bottle of red wine by the river. We went into cathedrals and churches, forever pulled by our Catholic guilt; she was chased from one by monks for wearing a skirt. In Firenze we were told to go to YAB or YAG (You Are Beautiful, You Are Gay), opting for the former, whispering the password to get in. Despite knowing each other since we first started school in our oversized blazers, I was still too scared to tell her. We woke up in the morning, our room overlooking the Basilica of Santa Maria Novella, the green and white illuminated in spring light like the underside of a leaf, our very own room with a view.

There were weekends spent in Bologna with a group of lesbians that I'd made friends with, all sporting rings on their left thumbs. I had never met so many queer people let alone known that there could be groups of friends who were queer. We danced until late as we spun to music clutching gin and tonics. I went down to Rome to stay with a friend of theirs. He showed me the city, we had beers at a gay bar, walked along the Tiber and listened to ghosts call from the Forum ruins. We went down to Naples and Pompeii. It was full of people frozen in time, husks and shells of their final moments, clinging to their loved ones. Whereas I felt like I was beginning to slowly come out of my own shell. The buildings and myths and sediments of history from my childhood shedding away. He taught me to twirl spaghetti properly under strip lights and darkness as we ate and waited for the train back to Rome. When we pulled into Termini station, we stood up and faced each other. He was getting off and I was taking the overnight train back home.

As the train doors slid shut, I realised I had closed the doors on my old life. I allowed myself to finally live out my own narrative. I got taken up into the hills where we sat on wood stumps and watched the sunrise over glasses of wine. I didn't know it was a date, or he was gay, until my housemate told me. I went on more dates and had sex with other guys, allowing myself the opportunity to explore myself, to change the narrative I had been given. I'd stopped exercising for the first time since I was a kid and lost all my muscle, my body no longer sculpted. I dropped to around 8 stone and let my hair grow out into a curly mess. I stopped trying to find myself in reflections, no longer scared of who and what stared back. No longer worried about what people thought of me because they all knew.

It was the first time in my life where I stopped. I could just be me. Not the high achiever sitting in front of his head of sixth form tearing my skin off my fingers as he asked why I wasn't applying to Oxford or Cambridge, not the sports star, not the heterosexual council estate kid. I'd been sprinting my whole life and this was the first time I could forget about the pressures, the expectations, the questions. My entire life I'd been living a different version of myself, living someone else's story. Yet in that city over 800 miles from home it didn't matter who I was or where I came from. No one cared and nor did I. The thing inside me was no longer an imposter, he – I – could live freely. I could stop pretending. I was just a person, just Michael, no longer being shoved into boxes, society's paradigms or my own internal prisons.

Before the summer was over, I booked flights to go stay with one of my best friends from secondary school who had moved to Florida in Year 9; and to see my brother who was stationed on the Pensacola. I left crying as my friend waved to me from the platform. I texted her that I couldn't do it, I shouldn't have booked the flights, this was my home. I'd finally been in a place where my sexuality and class didn't matter, where I wasn't scared of how someone would react to me being gay, where I could walk through history every day and leave my own behind.

In the blaze of Florida's summer, I hooked up a job at a clothes shop pretty quickly, the manager saying my English accent would boost their sales. Money was running even lower so I'd savour a $1 taco from Taco Bell that would last me the whole day. We'd drive from shopping mall to shopping mall with the air con blasting to try to break the wall of humidity that hit us each time we got out. One foot out the open window, the other resting on the dashboard as the anthem of our summer, 'We Didn't Start the Fire', played from the speakers as we sipped from $1 XXL sodas from McDonald's. The tarmac shimmered in the heat as we drove past people swinging signs to grab your attention, peeling off their baseball caps to wipe away button-sized sweat beads, lifting sunglasses to unearth hollow eyes. Spanish moss and shadows dripped from trees. We carried a boom box with us to play music in car parks as we roller-skated through the sunset around SUVs and trucks, gliding and dipping backwards to the beat of the CDs.

Glowing fast-food joints dotting the highways, neon signs pinging, the golden gloop of oil boiling, identical burgers being cut, the American dream wrapped up in branded paper. The shimmer of heat and sweat on the chests and arms of women pacing up and down Orange Blossom Trail in glittering dresses, frayed hot pants, t-shirts tied up in a knot, like we did as kids, while they twirled in the dust storms. The smear of make-up as it leaked from broken cupid bows. Waiting for a man, waiting for a dollar. In the wing mirrors signs were spun, this way, you need to go this way, to the horizon and the setting sun for the American dream. It wasn't to be my dream; it was my Americana shadow-life if we'd stayed living in the States. A parallel life, one of the many that happens if a different choice had been made, a different risk taken. I'd made mine, to return home for university.

We stood outside in the queue, wrapped up in scarves and gloves. The dark sea roaring behind us, the throb of the music from the club upstairs. My friends clutched cigarettes and each other, laughing and chatting, as we inched closer to the doorway. I looked around, scared in case someone I knew saw me, picking the skin around my fingers, shuffling on the spot. Wanting to get in but wanting to go home, too. The pink neon sign blazed above us, 'Revenge', the rainbow flags caught in the coastal winds. I'd never been to a gay club before, wondering whether this was the revenge of my heterosexuality, thrusting myself into a scene I didn't know and had never belonged to. Not knowing what upstairs would hold, how to act, if I'd fit in.

The lights cut me in pink and red and green and blue. Imprinting neon at the back of my eyes, we dripped in neon. The squash of flesh against mine, the flicker of glitter on bodies, the twirling and writhing to the beat of the music. Gaga blared out, claws up in the air to the chant of 'Ra, ra, ooh la la'. Every single person dressed and lived out who they were from crop tops, harnesses, short-shorts. Everyone screaming to Spice Girls, Britney, Beyoncé, Nelly Furtado, P!nk, Whitney, Shakira, Florence, every damn incredible woman that I'd loved as a kid. The music we had loved growing up, and been bullied for playing, in one place with hundreds of people. I'd found my home. We'd finally found where we belonged, found other people like us. This was my place; these were my people.

The gay world has its own set of rules, structures, tastes and behaviour. I was branded a 'gayby' by my friends as I'd not long come out and knew nothing about the scene. I didn't know what twinks or twunks, bears and daddies were. I didn't get the obsession with jockstraps; I wore them for lacrosse and they were uncomfortable and itchy. I couldn't read the signals and the cues. There was no guide so I learned by embracing everyone, my sexuality. It was normal here; this was a space I could finally be me.

I made a world in my own image: artists, singers, performance artists, queer friends where we created, opened up new spaces in our minds and made safe spaces. We sat on the floor singing along to a guitar with the window wide open and the inky sea out on the horizon. The piano in the corner with candelabras screwed in, wax dripping down the stick, as we created a chorus with glasses in our hands. Tracy Chapman, Amy MacDonald, 'The Passenger', Edith Piaf were the soundtracks of our evenings. Wine glasses were filled and emptied, lips stained, cigarettes squashed in scallop shells. We spent evenings curled up on sofas talking about our crushes, debating politics and art and performance and philosophy. We went to house parties, an *Alice in Wonderland* themed one with a room full of shishas and a guy dressed as the caterpillar, people rollerblading around the house with cupcakes iced with 'Eat me'. Performance art nights where strawberries were sliced into vaginas with a knife, pigs hearts carried in jars and a room flooded with refugees stranded on pallets. The marginalised have to find their sanctuaries and I found mine with these beautiful people who expressed themselves in so many different ways.

Even though I found my chosen family, ignorance still thrived even away at university where I thought who I was wouldn't matter.

How can you come from a council estate? You're well spoken, articulate, intelligent, I was asked over dinner. This type of comment wasn't unusual. I was told that working-class people who didn't go to university were lazy. It baffled them how someone who was working class could possibly go to university or not speak like a 'chav'. Somehow, given all their money and private education and privilege, they weren't educated out of ignorance.

Unlike them, I was there to push and expand my mind. I read Literature and fulfilled my dream of studying books from across time and the present, different cultures and sexualities and genders. I found books and ideas that I'd never had access to before or even believed could have been written. I took creative writing classes and I spent evenings in cafes filling up notebooks with short stories listening to Florence + the Machine, Lykke Li and Regina Spektor while the sea slowly became black. I was published, had my work used at performance nights. I fell asleep with the lights and my glasses still on, curled up with the open books around me. As I continued to open myself up and live and learn in new ways that I hadn't done previously, it opened up something else inside that'd been locked away.

A darkness was swelling, a tide that was pulling me into something deep and dark and terrible. I could feel the pain and the hurt and the trauma from my childhood start to drown me from the inside out, gurgling out from my mouth. The bottle I had sealed it in and thrown out to the sea of my subconscious was beginning to break and the words from the letter inside were seeping out. I was cracking. I couldn't block it anymore and I didn't know what to do.

At night, I stared into the darkness. Unable to sleep, unable to shut out the voices in my head as every morning I lay in bed watching the sun rise and the seagulls cry yet the shadows and night inside didn't disappear with the dawning light. It was late and something was tugging and pulling at me. I left the house, following a string that took me through the labyrinthine Lanes. People and laughter filled out the streets, I felt empty and alone as I was kept walking.

The pebbles crunched under my shoes, wet and black and glinting in the moonlight. The sea in front of me a black mirror, as if the sky had collapsed onto its surface. The carcass of the burned old pier collapsing – a dark gash in the horizon. The pier's lights tossed up and drowning in the sea. It was empty and vast and dark yet full and turbulent and uncontrollable. I stood in the shore, my feet wet. It was inviting, calling out to me. The siren inside calling me to it. There was a face in the water that collided with my own. My reflection fragments in the waves. Split and thrashed around. Overwhelmed by the power of the night around me and the darkness it was pulling me towards. Some force that wanted me to keep going further. I walked deeper into the waters, the place where so many things begin, and where I wanted everything to end.

Something stopped me. I stepped back on the shore and sat down and started crying. I called a friend who luckily answered despite it being so late.

'Mike, are you okay?'

'No, I'm not okay.' Finally saying those words, admitting out loud that I wasn't and I needed help was a release I hadn't realised I needed. For years I'd been suppressing so much that had happened to me, and it had finally broken free. I'd talked to friends, sought their advice, but it was rarely about my past. The past was the past, it didn't matter. I didn't understand that the past influenced the present and could change the future for good or bad. My mind had gotten to the point where it couldn't take it anymore and I'd reached the point where I could no longer ignore what I was going through.

I ended up going to therapy, which was the first time I talked properly about my childhood, acknowledged what happened, sought help to try to stitch together the broken parts. Six weeks doesn't cure a childhood. I thought I'd been fixed, but it wasn't about being 'fixed', it was about recognising and understanding what had happened in order to move forward.

The years of containing a secret, hiding who I really was, waking up and pretending to be someone else, wearing a skin that didn't belong to me is scarring. Shame, while I didn't feel its latent presence, was embedded in my DNA, an unknown chromosome that exerted its influence and affected everything about me. Coming out, whether to friends or family, doesn't eradicate the past and what has happened.

Coming out isn't the end but the beginning of the journey to becoming who you are and understanding how you got there. I've learned that being gay isn't a switch, it's a process and a journey. I spent over eighteen years hiding, denying, shaming myself for the person that was trapped in a body. My gay self had been living in a state of stasis for that same duration: isolated, locked up, starving. I'd been trying to walk and run in a life that wasn't mine and there was the expectancy that once you come out or accept your sexuality you sprint into fully fledged queerness just from the act of voicing it.

Shame doesn't shed easily. It's not something that you peel off at the end of the day and place in the closet and throw back on when you feel like it. It's grafted on and in you. The conditioning we receive from others and society, and the conditioning we put ourselves through in order to survive, doesn't dissolve once we come out of the proverbial closet. It's a reckoning I, so many of us, face on a daily basis. Reinforcing to ourselves that we are normal, we deserve the best, that we can get through another day. It can consume if not handled carefully.

A 2021 survey by Stonewall found that 84 per cent of students were more likely to be more open about their sexuality and gender identity when going to higher education. They also found that queer students were four times more likely to declare a mental health condition.[1] This shows that while university or moving away from home allows more freedom and acceptance, there is an impact on our mental health that we carry from childhood that needs support and attention. Leaving home is not end game – it's the beginning of many journeys. It won't solve the issues of abuse, trauma and bullying experienced in adolescence. Finding allies and a place that is home are an important step but so is identifying and acknowledging the issues from before. I bottled it up and stored it away, and then once it was full it cracked.

Italy and university provided me with the opportunity to be myself. Different skies, different streets, different people. They played a crucial role in my development not only into adulthood but into my sexuality. Back home, I didn't feel I could be myself or that self would be accepted. There weren't the variety of masculinities, sexualities, genders that I could identify with, in which I could see myself reflected. Brighton and Italy gave me the space, the time, the community, the opportunity to discover who I was.

Leaving home is a crucial point for so many people in their journey to accepting who they are, finding a home, creating a chosen family. A space where you can freely express yourself without fear or judgement is crucial. Moving from the rural to the urban was vital for me: it gave me freedom and anonymity and the opportunity to find a scene and similar people or allies. The urban gave me a different belonging that I didn't have in the rural space. Studies have found that rural constructs of gender are narrow and traditional[2] thus making it difficult for queer people who do not conform to those narratives. Migration to the urban allows queer people to find people and constructs and spaces that they can't find back in the countryside.

My journey is not every journey, you have to find the place you call home and where you belong. This doesn't have to be a city or a university, it can be a hamlet, where you grew up, the seaside, a different country – as long as you have support and safety. I miss the countryside; I miss the silence and the memories and the comfort. Often as a kid I would sing 'Go The Distance' from Disney's *Hercules* and dream about a place beyond the horizon where I belonged. I craved somewhere else, knew I belonged someplace else. I needed art and theatre, music and motion, different cultures and peoples that my hometown, and the estate, couldn't provide. If you can't move away, find connections in whatever way you can: social media, concerts, book groups, forums. Belonging, and home, are evolving. People move, relationships break up, new ones are found, different friendship groups are made. I found a new home and myself, but it didn't help me escape what I'd been suppressing, it didn't help me understand how so much of it had been founded in adolescence. The trauma, bullying and abuse we go through before we reach adulthood needs to be supported properly by institutions to avoid situations of depression or suicide and other mental health conditions. My university time was fundamental to my opening up, my acceptance and understanding, so different to my school days where I was silently gagged by laws and societal structures unknown to me at the time.

I didn't realise at the time that this wasn't the end of reckoning with my mental health and demons. It was just the beginning of the journey.

Chapter Nine

Hundreds of students ran and screamed down the corridor as I walked through the Georgian building. Stained glass windows with roses twining around the panes, portraits, a hidden stairwell nicknamed Platform 9¾. Out on the fields, girls swooped and dived for flying balls like they were playing Quidditch, which I learned was a sport called lacrosse. My blazer's sleeves hid my hands, my green and purple tie done perfectly by my mum. Shirt crisp and ironed, the red badge on my chest indicating my new house, where I belonged. I'd gone from a small village primary school with nine of us in my year to the former grammar school in town. It had two sites and centuries of history. It was a world so far-flung from what I knew.

I'd decided not to go to the local comprehensive in the village near the estate where my best friend from primary school had gone. The thought of spending another five years with the people who bullied me wasn't an option. At least if I had gone somewhere else, this time round I'd only have to deal with them when out on the estate. They soon found new ways to bully me as I went to the 'posh' school.

'Did you have cucumber sandwiches and tea at school today?' They asked when out on the green.

'Yeah, we get detention if we don't have our pinkies out,' I replied. They told me I now spoke posh, I lived on the 'posh side' of the estate. There were always differences to be found, hierarchies that had to be asserted. I was no longer one of them, which I was fine with.

Secondary school was the place where I was given the chance to rebrand. My past was left behind and I could be who I wanted. I wasn't the Billy Elliot of the estate, nor was I the council estate kid. I kept those things closely guarded. There was an intrinsic fear of revealing too much about myself and where I came from after what I experienced in primary school. Once bitten, twice shy. The wounds were still fresh, easy to open back up. The divisions and differences I had learned on the estate, and at primary school, were just as present here.

I'd escaped the kids on the estate in the day, but it became increasingly clear that I didn't belong at my new school. There were new rules and structures to understand and navigate. They had parents and grandparents who went to university, first and second and third homes, their holidays were spent skiing down mountains. The difference was clear in the foods they ate, the words they knew, the primary schools they went to that actually invested and believed in them. These weren't council estate kids; this was a different game. I soon felt forced to assimilate and be like them: the way they spoke, the way they interacted, the reference points. Slipping into a new body, shifting the root of my tongue so I sounded, looked, like them.

Pessimism and self-doubt were an inheritance I took with me. I didn't know that this was something called imposter syndrome. But no one at my new school knew anything about me. It allowed me to escape from the old me and create a new persona. It was my opportunity to erase the past and create an easier future. Create the myth and narrative, build the story for people to believe. Erase the common out of me. Fake it until you make it. New chapter, new story, new me.

I soon learned that once the civilised masks were peeled off, the wealthier kids were no different. Lockers were pushed in front of the classroom door so the teacher couldn't get in, food fights and eruptions of flame as a gas tap was set on fire. I saw chunks of hair ripped from a scalp, blood spatter on blouses, a guy hit another with a hockey stick, the fights organised between groups for after school on the field. Working-class people are often depicted as being violent delinquents with no desire to better ourselves or learn. Violence, aggression, the rejection of education, is not confined to the working class. School soon taught me that money didn't make you better. It gave you more opportunities, it gave you the belief that you were better. We were given a stigma to battle through to be accepted and be taken seriously. They were no different to me or the kids on the estate. The difference was the world had told them they were better.

There was an easiness to so many of them. A privilege, they belonged, it all came so naturally to them. They had a blueprint to follow. Getting good grades was my one ticket to getting out of the estate. My parents constantly reinforced the importance of doing well at school and made sure we did. Gymnastics was taken from me so education had to be my plan B. One girl told me that my competitiveness was my most unattractive quality. I had to be competitive because chances weren't going to fall in my lap. I had to make them. To prove that I was worth something and better than what people had thought of me. To be someone when I'd been told I was a no one by others.

Once, I was sitting in the common room studying with a friend. She put down her pen and looked at me.

'Why do you always work so hard?'

'Because I have to,' I replied, without looking up from my book. Because I had to work ten times harder. There was no room for error. I threw myself into my education. I made sure I excelled in everything: deputy house captain, co-writing the play for the house drama competition, top grades, additional qualifications, on the 'gifted and talented list' for creative writing. Overachieving is a way for people who have been through shame-based trauma to try 'to meet unreachable standards in order to gain the acceptance of others'.[1] In abusive relationships this need to gain acceptance, to overachieve to seem good in the abuser's eyes, while at the same time never feeling good enough, can be wielded to control the abusee. Overachieving was where I found my validation, if I couldn't find validity for my hidden identities.

Unlike in primary school, my work and talent were appreciated and invested in by some of my teachers. English had always been my best subject, but secondary school was really where I flourished. I wrote short stories and poems that I filled with my angst and worries. I created new worlds of powerful women and hidden secrets. Yet, there were times when some teachers and classmates questioned whether it was my work or how I knew specific vocabulary. As if someone from my station couldn't have produced something like that. It was because I always pushed myself to be better, my parents made sure we did our homework, did extra reading, and yet somehow doing well was something I was being made to feel guilty for or like I hadn't earned it myself.

My GCSE and A Level English teachers were the game changers. They encouraged my creative writing, spoke to me about my future, if I'd read English at university, what my options were. Making suggestions about books to read, how to make my work better. They believed in me and in my abilities. The belief and investment from a teacher can be transformative. Once, after class, I spoke with one of my teachers expressing my worry about whether I'd get the grade I wanted, whether my work was good enough. I always needed and felt I had to be better, the best.

'Mike, you're one of the most tenacious students I've taught. You'll be absolutely fine,' she told me. It was that tenacity to do well, my tenacity to survive that I got from my parents and the estate, that helped me excel. I would get there, no matter what. I truly must thank them for changing the direction of my life. Without their dedication and excellent teaching, I don't know what I would be doing. They gave me the powerful gift of belief when teachers from as early as the age of 5 made sure I didn't believe in myself because I came from an estate. It planted a seed inside that would bloom and grow, and when more often than not I doubted myself and my ability to succeed, they reminded me that I could.

My first poem was published in a pamphlet when I was 17. It was about apples and mirrors, hiding and reflecting yourself, a fall from grace. I walked into the sixth form common room and someone had written it in marker across the walls. They laughed and laughed. *So gay. How can you ever be a writer? Is this a joke?* Just like so many other things in my life thus far, I had to defend myself. I was put back in my place, told not to be ambitious, made to feel ashamed because my interests weren't what aligned with 'traditional' male interests.

I felt like once again I was being pushed back into that box my primary school teachers put me in, just another council estate skank. How could the council estate kid become a writer? I'd done everything I could to fit in, to align myself with how they were. It was never enough. I'd always feel inadequate compared with them and the lives they had. I was waiting, biding my time to be revealed as a fraud. They belonged in a world and it fostered confidence in them; we'd been trained the opposite. If they'd read between the lines of the imagery in that poem, they probably would have understood what I was trying to tell the world behind those metaphors.

The tiles were shiny with steam. Ties whipped at flesh trying its best to rid itself of childhood. Lynx-scented mushroom clouds erupted across the changing room. Bodies twisted and curled as they clung to clothes and damp towels. Too ashamed of what was hidden underneath, even though it was what they staked their status on. The shrill laughter echoed like a nursery rhyme from a childhood long ago as trousers were hurriedly pulled up after someone was spotted who hadn't graduated from pants to boxers. I kept my eyes firmly fixed on the hooks.

The changing rooms were the epicentre of testosterone. Where sweat and dirt clung to surfaces, flesh and inorganic, football boots smashed against the wall to get clods of dirt out, chants breaking out, the cool kids peacocking. It was feral and carnal and suffocating. The bodies that were growing and morphing, skin stretching and muscle twining. While the masculinity on the estate was intense, it was never in this close proximity, where you had to unveil and assert your manhood every day. We'd moved from learning about how to join the club to making sure we belonged in it. There was no other place more rigid in those structures than the changing rooms.

There was a thud. Everyone stopped and looked at a book flat open in the puddles on the floor absorbing the dirt and sweat into the pages.

'Dropped your gay card, mate,' someone shouted. The laughter followed as he stuffed the damp book back in his bag. They branded him 'book boy' for a while. I suppose they had learned what alliteration was. School was an obstacle course and an ever-updating list of things you had to navigate, learn and hide in order not to be branded 'gay'. Books, writing, subjects, ways of walking, ways of talking, music, which shows you watched – the list was infinite. The result always the same. I'd learned years before in primary school not to let anything that may give the whiff of queer be known to other guys. Reading and writing were two of them. On the weekends I'd scuttle down the high street glancing over my shoulder, scanning the groups of people to make sure I didn't know anyone before slipping into Waterstones or the library. The same ritual was performed on the way out with the bag of books folded up and placed under my arm so even if I did bump into someone, they wouldn't know what I had bought.

Gay was something not to be associated with. *You're gay, that's gay, it's gay, so gay, don't be gay.* It was used for everything and anything, pair it in any combination, in any type of clause, team it up with other swearwords. It really was quite the versatile word. It was always a pejorative. That word was enough to terrify most of us. All it took was to be called it once for your social status, your credibility, your manhood to be derailed. No one wanted to be branded as the 'gay kid'. One girl in Year 9 came out as bisexual. She was eradicated for it. I should have defended her, been an ally, but I was too scared to relive what I'd gone through in primary school. Queerness wasn't something that was talked about in class, it wasn't something positive, it was something that wasn't acceptable. It was a threat and an insult.

One summer afternoon, the guys in my year were summoned to the sports hall without any explanation. There were shuffles, eyes flitting at each other, laughter and shouts of, *We're in for it now, boys!* Once we'd all sat down cross-legged or legs splayed, depending how you asserted yourself, two of the science teachers walked to the front.

'What's in your wallet?' one shouted, the catchphrase from that credit card advert, as he whipped out a dildo from his blazer. Everyone laughed as expected from a group of 14-year-old boys.

'Time for some sex education,' he said over the giggles and shoving of shoulders as people were accused of using one. He certainly broke the ice to broach a subject all teachers must hate giving to hundreds of teenage boys whose hormones were vibrating and just about everything else pulsing. They asked us to write down one question to put in a bowl for them to answer. The previous sex education lessons we'd received were purely looking at anatomical drawings of genitalia, how to get someone pregnant and how not to. They were giving us the opportunity to ask what we needed to know. Man to man.

There were five minutes to think about what we needed to ask and scribble it down. Some people did it together, whispering in each other's ears, concocting up something to ask, others sweated and flushed, others threw their paper to the side. Once the last paper had been gathered there was a notable shift in the energy. Waiting, tense, looking around. People were scared that their question may be identified.

'Will eleven inches be too big for someone?' The teachers sagged at the inevitable size question. They made their way through answering each one either using science or their own experience. It was an open way to discuss our fears and curiosities to make us more aware about our bodies, relationships and sex. It was a way to open a dialogue about the personal that so many guys felt difficult doing. It made it a collective experience and normalised what was happening in our lives as we were changing. We're all the same so we shouldn't feel ashamed.

'How do I know if I'm gay?'

We weren't all the same. The teachers looked at each other awkwardly. Hundreds of eyes looked around, murmurs, laughter, whispers. *Queer, batty, poof.* The lullaby of my childhood rippled through the air. Someone amongst the ranks had broken formation. People shuffled, looking around to see if they could decipher who had written those forbidden words. The silence lurked. It throbbed and grew. Punctuated each and every one of us in case we were accused, in case we were, in case it was true. A primordial terror.

'You just know,' one of the teachers answered. Clearly neither had experienced it or had the scientific reasons they relied on before. In that hall there was a lost soul, a queer soul drowning amongst the sea of perceived heterosexual boys, needing a lifejacket to be thrown out. Someone was brave enough to reach out and try to find the reassurance they needed. To find validation about what they were feeling. Yet, there was no elaboration from either of them. No attempt to say this was normal, to offer information from elsewhere that could have given them guidance. There was no coda following those words to say, 'Which is okay. Some people are gay, get over it.' Instead, his hand shot back in the bowl to whip out another question.

As the others laughed, I looked down at the floor and tried to shrink myself or avoid making eye contact with anyone else. Suddenly the summer heat, the temperature in the hall was rising, my cheeks flushing. I thought if they looked at me, they would see the guilt stirring there. I picked at my nails, tugging and pulling flesh until blood dripped down my fingers. I wanted it to be over, it'd all been fun and games until then. Move onto a new question, wrap it up, send us out for lunch.

Deep down, it was the question I wish I had asked and wish I had known the answer to. While I may have suspected before, it was at this age that I started to fully understand and fully fear what I may have been. My eyes lingering on the contours of faces, the shift of muscle, the streaks of stubble. I didn't realise it was a crush or attraction. I didn't know other gay people, I'd never seen it, I didn't understand myself. I'd had a few two-week whirlwind girlfriends where we passed notes to each other and met up in town on the weekend. We're born into a world that is built for us to be, and assumes that we are, heterosexual, so I did it too: fell in line, followed the script. But there was a shadow expanding inside that wouldn't disappear. Some feeling that was lurking that I wasn't attracted to girls, I just enjoyed hanging out with them. I'd done all I could to mask it, but something was stirring inside me and there was no outlet for me to explore it, understand it, for it to be confirmed.

Answering that question scrawled hurriedly on a little piece of paper could have given so many people in that hall the confirmation that they were normal, and to normalise it to those who weren't. It could have given me confirmation. They had the opportunity to try and stop the homophobic taunts used as everyday language. That opportunity was swept under the carpet, locked in the closet. It put so many of us back in. It wasn't my question. I wouldn't have dared. Eat your words, eat your soul. Out of sight, out of mind. If it's not voiced, it doesn't exist.

Someone in that hall was brave enough to try find out the answer, but their cries fell on deaf ears. I didn't have the courage to reach out, to try and understand what those feelings were. Part of me wished to know who it was so we could talk, be friends, figure it out together. Even if I had known, I wasn't at the point where I had accepted it myself. It would have been death by association. Neither he, nor I, came out publicly during school. I hope he has now, I hope he's had his questions answered, I hope he's doing okay.

The word gay was constantly used negatively; however, it was the one thing that wasn't present in school. Not in books, not in class discussions, not in sex education, or literature, or biology or history, not in personal development. It didn't exist. It was some mythic, dangerous thing that was never to be discussed or acknowledged, swept under the carpet. Except as an insult. That was 2004, only a year had passed since Section 28 had been repealed after a fifteen-year reign of terror.

I'd never heard of it before, hadn't seen it in the news and it would be years until I learned what it was. Something doesn't need to be known for its damage to be felt. Through the silence it enforced, I certainly felt its destruction. The amendment was enacted in 1988 at the height of the AIDS epidemic when the gay community needed support the most. It was a horrific attempt to supress a minority already struggling to find equality and acceptance in a country where 75 per cent of the country thought homosexuality was wrong.[2]

It prohibited local authorities and schools from teaching and promoting the acceptability of homosexuality or providing resources, support or services to the LGBTQ+ community. Through this gagging order countless young queer people were left underprepared to enter adulthood with the necessary resources and education to prepare them. It left generations of young people without ever being able to be taught or recognised that they were normal. It was a way to reinforce 'traditional morals' and avoid 'corrupting' children with homosexuality, or, in Thatcher's own words, that they are being taught that they have the 'inalienable right to be gay'. In other words, our sexualities are a thing that can be taken away, they don't belong to us, it's a choice. We don't belong in this society. There is no love for us.

The sex education we were taught was all within the heterosexual matrix. How men and women have sex, what is a healthy relationship between men and women, what is rape in the context of men and women, what does 'no' mean in the context of men and women, how to avoid getting pregnant, how pregnancy works, how STIs are transmitted between men and women, what is love and affection between men and women, how to be safe on a night out for women, how to be a decent man towards women. I read the books and did the homework on all these things. It confirmed and reflected the heterosexual world with no room for anyone else.

We weren't taught what a healthy same-gender relationship is, about safe sex between men, about douching or how lubricant should be used during anal sex to avoid condoms breaking, that men can love each other and can hug and kiss and show affection. It stopped us learning that men can be abused physically, sexually, mentally and emotionally. We weren't taught about consent. Only one in five queer students learn about safe sex and contraception at school.[3] It would have taught us the power to say 'no' and create boundaries to protect ourselves. Gay or lesbian or bi or trans or queer were never said. We were never acknowledged. Left unaware that other people were out there just like us. It was another lesson in feeling worthless and abnormal.

We weren't taught how to come out, when to come out, where to come out. The support available for when you do. It could have saved lives. Instead, people – I – suffered in silence, bearing a struggle, self-hatred, confusion and unknowing that ate and consumed and festered and rotted me. If Section 28 had never existed, maybe that boy's question during that assembly would have been answered, those teachers would have been prepared and comfortable to teach what needs to be taught.

That boy could have walked away feeling proud of who he is, I could have walked away with a bit more confidence to accept who I was rather than burying it deeper. Instead, it silenced. We were not saved but starved and it sent us into adulthood helpless when confronted with dangerous situations and relationships. We were abandoned to haul our mental health conditions into adulthood, to not understand that same-gender abuse can happen, to be primed to believe that abusive or toxic relationships are normal.

Section 28 is a silent killer. Homophobia seeks to destroy and supress, and Section 28 helped to facilitate the self-destruction of so many queer people. It had done its job. This legislation didn't save us, it choked us. It left me underprepared, gasping, drowning, starved for answers, dignity, validation that left me stumbling into adulthood with no knowledge of the gay world I would enter. Some never would. The underdeveloped self-worth from years of bullying, from years of not knowing if I was normal, from years of fear led me down an untrodden shadowed path where self-destruction lurked.

It's pushed many to substance abuse, toxic relationships, abusive relationships, while living with poor mental health and self-esteem. It's pushed people to find that validation, even if just for a moment, in unhealthy and dangerous ways to destroy and eradicate the hate and shame they feel. Or for a minute to feel connected or loved by someone. Thatcher thought that Section 28 would save young people, but little did I know that as a boy with his legs crossed and a big secret that this was what I had waiting for me, this would be the consequence.

I wish that there had been one person who had told me about the incredible people I would meet: the chosen family, the ones who will love us, the people who would literally and figuratively pick you up and keep you going when you finally shatter, that it would be okay when I came out to my family. The ones who would make the pain and trauma of childhood worth it as you're cuddled up together on the sofa watching a film with someone just like you or dancing until dawn. Finally belonging, finally accepted. About the courage and strength and bravery our ancestors had to fight for decriminalisation and equality. I wish I had been taught that someday I would be proud of who I am and the community I belong to. Not to minimise and hide and be scared of who I was. I wish I had been taught to go to the police. To report abuse from strangers, colleagues, lovers. It couldn't happen because it didn't exist. We were men and it doesn't happen to men.

The simple confirmation that being queer is normal could have been enough. Those simple words, without even anything else, could have been enough to save lives, to save years of self-torment and hate, avoiding the epidemic of mental health problems in the community. It could've had the power to let someone know that they deserve love, to love themselves, they have worth. Fostering a healthy relationship with themselves and someone else could be possible.

Out in the countryside the ivy and the trees and the darkness grew thicker and denser, closing in around me. Pushed further and further into my head, rejecting, hating and not understanding the transformation that was happening inside me. It was a metamorphosis I didn't want; I didn't understand that it was something beautiful. The question was asked, the question was rejected. The world rejected a reflection and confirmation of who I was. I was denied the ability to understand about the incredible sensations, and people, and love that would come. Instead, it reinforced the poor self-esteem that had already been conditioned into me. It would help drive me into a world full of danger that I never knew was possible.

In one survey, 86 per cent of secondary school teachers stated that students they teach have experienced homophobia,[4] and 43 per cent of LGBT students said they aren't able to be their true selves at school.[5] Sadly, 18 per cent of those bullied haven't told anyone about it,[6] just like I didn't in primary school, out of fear or because they don't feel the world around them will support or accept them. The bullying and othering LGBTQ+ people face during adolescence instils shame in us, it instils self-hatred toward our identity so much so that LGBT+ youth are twice as likely to consider suicide, rising to three times for Black LGBT+ young people.[7] We enter adulthood without feeling normal or accepted, without a validated identity impacting our self-esteem, confidence and self-worth translating into a multitude of mental health problems. In fact, one in three mental health conditions in adulthood correspond to childhood trauma.[8] How much of our mental health problems as queer people correspond with the bullying and vacuum of support and representation in adolescence?

No doubt even since I left school in 2008 things have improved. There are more inclusive books, TV shows and films or social media to find other queer people. There are charities such as Diversity Role Models who send people into schools to teach about inclusion and diversity and see reflections of themselves. In fact, positive LGBTQ+ messaging sees a drop of 9 per cent in young queer people contemplating suicide and 5 per cent for non-LGBTQ+ people.[9] Their work, in the absence of the government interventions, is essential to ensure that young people feel accepted, foster diversity and find the support they need when beginning to understand their sexuality or identity.

In 2019, legislation was passed so that schools must include teaching about LGBTQ+ sex and relationships from September 2020. This is a landmark achievement that will give so many young people questioning their gender and sexuality the hope and understanding of who they are, hopefully leaving school with a greater self-respect and self-worth than I did. With more inclusive education and better resources, the bullying we faced growing up could have been better handled by educators. Inclusive education can help reduce bullying and break down phobias, discrimination and stigmas. It's also vital in combatting queerphobic bullying, breaking down prejudices and creating allies. It can stop the shame, the internalised hate and homophobia that continue to stick to us as adults.

Yet, because of this victory, there were protests by parents in Birmingham in 2019 against LGBTQ+ inclusive education that took a High Court order to ban them. It's against religious teachings, it's against natural law, I don't want it to make my child queer, I don't want it to corrupt them, they're too young to learn about this, it breaks down family traditions and values, what on earth will they be taught next? It harks back to Thatcher.

In March 2020, the Conservative government defunded anti-bullying initiatives. It's been over two years since they pledged to ban conversion therapy, which amounts to torture, and they have since announced in 2022 that it will exclude our trans siblings. In fact, 26 per cent of doctors in 2021 refused to support the British Medical Association lobbying to ban conversion therapy. We are not out of the woods yet to ensure that young people get the teaching and support they need.

The impact of Section 28 still lingers, the complacency by each government since to rectify its damage shows in how queer youth feel today. LGBTQ+ charity Just Like Us reports that LGBT+ young people are twice as likely to have depression, anxiety and panic attacks. They are three times as likely to self-harm and twice as likely to consider suicide.[10] These figures are from 2021, eighteen years since Section 28 was repealed. Despite all the advances, society is still geared up to other queer people, the impact on mental health is profound, this adversity and pain we face in adolescence is carried through to adulthood where it continues to wreak havoc in our daily lives and relationships.

It once again shows that there are people out there who wish to suffocate young people, to deny them the right to understand who they are and learn about queer history. It also stops the education of heterosexual young people which would help avoid the queerphobic bullying that damages our mental health and worth. If those protestors had had inclusive education when they were young, perhaps it never would have been an issue. Charities and independent organisations can only do so much. The Department of Education needs to deliver better resources, support and education to schools and education practitioners.

I've spoken with friends, queer and heterosexual alike, and people older and younger than me who were kind enough to open up about their experiences. No one remembers or had an inclusive queer education. I've spoken with teachers who have said despite Section 28 being removed and the implementation of the new law, LGBTQ+ inclusive education is still minimal. 86 per cent of primary teachers have received no training on how to tackle homophobic bullying.[11] The resources and knowledge of what queer people need to be taught is rudimentary and doesn't prepare them in the same way. This shows the generational damage Section 28 has done, even to young people now, and the need for systemic change to turn the tide on preparing young people for adulthood. It's essential that young queer people are educated properly not only to help avoid mental health issues and self-destructive behaviour, but for them to have the opportunity to live freely and safely.

While being born in the 1990s gave me an enormous privilege compared with my predecessors who fought for my rights to be legal, and equal, there were still the ramifications of anti-queer policies and a lack of queer visibility and acceptance. Throughout school, I was trapped in a body and an existence that didn't belong to me knowing that I couldn't live that true self safely. Without knowing what I was feeling was normal, understanding what I was feeling. Suppression can lead to self-destruction. School isn't there just to teach us about subjects but to prepare us for adulthood, which should be inclusive of relationships, heterosexual and queer, sex and consent.

Instead, I left school unprepared for the risks that lay ahead of me. I'd suppressed who I was, hated what I was, carrying the private battles of trauma, abuse, bullying into my adulthood. I left school vulnerable and unequipped about the queer world I would enter, how to protect myself, not knowing I could be abused, and the dangers that could come. I'd been trained to a heterosexual narrative. The world had set me up for a perfect storm. I was forced to run into a world I didn't know about. I was running towards danger without knowing what it looked like and how the damage done at school would be wielded to trap me in abuse.

Chapter Ten

Flesh slapped together. The grunts and pants and sighs. The drip dripping of sweat onto my face. I focused on the wall, finding the cracks, the tiny little fissures in the surface that if you pulled away the layers of paint you'd find deeper, darker wounds in the structure. He stared down at me, I stared back vacantly. Descending deeper into myself, pushing my consciousness away. Left my body empty, just a shell for him to use. Overriding my emotions, overriding attachment. Severed the bonds. Detached from the person in the bed with me. Detached from myself. When the door closed, it was another chapter closed. Full stop.

I walked along the Thames, not caring where I was going. Just following that thread through the city, leading me deeper into the labyrinth. The thousands of faces bumping past, laughing, places to get to, people to see. The networks and connections running beneath and around me, while I cut off the ones inside me. The wires and gears inside whirring, becoming something mechanical, just another cog in the system. Just another item to push off the conveyor belt of lust.

It's underneath the sheets and in the aftermath of gasps where we create fictions of ourselves. The narrative of our bodies. That was the narrative I gave my body: if someone craved it, I could find validation. I fuck therefore I am. I've held many hands, waited for many to come and lead me away.

I've felt so much flesh against mine that has disappeared. Comforted by the flash and blur of relentless bodies. Felt the ghostly remains as I slept under half-empty, loveless sheets. Just an echo of a memory, a dream of a body, the spectre of love. Pulling on clothes to try to cover the humiliation that was felt underneath the layers. That one moment gave me the validation that I needed, to be wanted just for a moment, to feel something for just a moment. To feel whole was something I desired. Curled up hoping one would want to stay a little longer. Hoping that I would find love, find it for myself.

I downloaded apps and internet dated. Met guys for drinks or dinner, going for walks or just hooking up. I was Pygmalion. Each day I sculpted lust, carved it from my imagination. Pictures get swapped, judged in a snap second, our bodies become virtual and physical currency. It shows us how much we're worth, valued by 2D lovers. They existed and morphed in the confines of my mind. Our lust moved along data, our passion flashing in pixels. I stopped the pursuit of love and instead offered up my body for sacrifice. Time is suspended in the virtual world of wantonness. There was no past, there was no present when we can erase our history. When we become scrapped data.

I graduated from Brighton into a different world and scene in London. Brighton felt like a bubble, wrapped up and safe. I was lost in this new city, consumed and overwhelmed. The country boy navigating through different lives and stories, towering buildings and shadowed alleys and bedrooms. So much choice, so many options. Always a choice, there's always another option. Which one should I choose? Roll the dice and see. I saw in others what I felt in myself. Looking for the same thing but not knowing what it was or how to get there. We were mirroring each other and not able to cross the glass. Something kept us separated from each other, from ourselves. Always looking for the other halves of ourselves.

We're promised love. From the moment we're born it's the first promise we're given. From our parents, from books, from films, from others. I'll love you forever. Just wait for love to happen. Love will come. There's someone for everyone. You'll meet your perfect match, one day. One day it will happen. We keep waiting, hoping, loving. A prince to save me, a princess to be saved. I reinvented love into sex and physicality. I couldn't find love for myself so I found the validation in the unhealthiest of ways: sex and alcohol. How many times do I have to reinvent love? As many as it takes.

London gave me anonymity. I could solely be a number, just another body out of the millions that passed through the Tube, through beds. I could find what I wanted. I could find the validation in who I was through my body. Sex and virility gave me validation of my masculinity and sexuality. It meant I was wanted. It, for a moment, squashed down the deep-rooted lack of self-esteem for who and what I was. Those hook-ups were a way to validate my own existence. To find validation for what I had always rejected. To try feel in control, to try claim control, to find acceptance even fleetingly so I wasn't worthless.

I didn't feel prepared for this type of lifestyle, where hooking-up was normal, where being disposable was normal. But I threw myself into it, I wanted to give up to that Dionysian side of me that I had buried so deep. Let out the chaos and the rage and the hunger and the craving. To explore, to experience different types of love and lust. I explored the Pit, drunk from the river Lethe to forget the hurt, the pain, the abuse. I found my ways to self-protect. One was to run from who I was, the other to destroy it. Stumbling in the darkness in an inevitable pursuit of destruction. So, I kept running.

Every morning the blare of my alarm would cut through the empty sleep. Shower, rinse off the grime and sweat and fog, change. The bubble of the macchinetta and the gold-frothed coffee gurgling out. Smoke on the way to the station, do my university reading on the 45-minute commute, smoke on the way from the station to work. Work for 8 hours, 45-minute commute back, coffee when I got home. Write until 3 a.m., up at 7 a.m. to go back to work. Write until 3 a.m., up at 7 a.m. for classes. Out for drinks, feed the dried-up darkness, house party, necking tinnies on the Tube before the next one. Keep dancing, keep moving, keep running, keep drinking. Wake up at 7 a.m., pour the coffee, keep going. I'd moved to London to do a masters where I was working full-time on top of it. Sliding from one to another, partying, writing, partying. My body was an engine and I fuelled it with nicotine and caffeine fumes, sweetened with the sugars from the alcohol my body churned.

Once I graduated, I got my first internship at a leading literary agency. The money they offered for working full-time wasn't even enough to cover rent let alone food or bills. Luckily, I had friends who lived in a big house in Vauxhall who said I could stay there while I did it. It was a spare room on the ground floor where there was a pull-down bed that acted as a partition from the other part of the room where their bikes were stored. It was a saving grace for me that I could stay with them and pay enough money that left me with some to actually live. It gave me the opportunity to do what I'd always wanted to do: work with books.

I stepped into that agency filled with wonder and fear and hope. Books lining the wall, manuscripts on desks, agents on phones to authors and editors, famous authors swooping in and out to discuss deals and foreign rights. The council estate boy had made it into the book world. That world where I read to escape felt so far-flung from this world of jumping on the Tube to go and give second opinions on submissions, making tea and coffee for authors whose work and words I'd poured over growing up. I had to book famous restaurants I'd never heard of, tables at Soho House without knowing why it was different to other houses in Soho.

When assisting the CEO for a week, in my first internship, one of the other agents came over to the desk and looked down at me.

'Why do you think you're good enough to work for her?' I was asked. We'd never spoken before and this was the only thing that was ever said between us. I didn't reply, what was there for me to say? I was trying to get by, doing my best to try and make it. I was definitely told that this wasn't where I belonged. I didn't think I was good enough, but I did my best to make sure no one knew that. Staying late, reading after work, asking for more work and more responsibility. I was living a dream; one I had never expected to realise. Not even knowing how to get into publishing, there was no blueprint, no precedent for me to follow. I'd figure it out, without trying to be figured out.

In between internships, I worked at a call centre for a fruit and veg company. I got free fruit and veg but was shouted at for bruised plums and missing boxes, called a charlatan and a liar by angry customers. I woke up at 5 a.m. on some days to get to the office, always keeping the end goal in mind that it was so I could afford to do another round of unpaid work experience.

To make sure that I would make it in publishing. Eventually, I got my break at a publishing house.

I edited anthologies, planned launch parties and came up with marketing ideas. I'd fill evenings and weekends with book and exhibition launches, literary events, performance art nights, meeting friends for drinks topped off with dancing until late. I'd triple, quadruple-book myself, sliding from Tube to platform, running up escalators, diving through closing doors, sighing as the stop button was pressed at every bus stop. The trill in my voice, *darling*, as I kissed cheeks, slapped backs, hugged tightly. I kept running, kept moving, kept myself busy so I would never stop to have to think.

I twirled in the darkness, pumped with jabbing lights of blue, green, red, yellow. Spots of white swirling across the floor, the ceiling, my body. I swayed on top of a pool table, clutching a drink in one hand, the other thrust in the air as I slid my body up and down. The stage where I'd earlier belted out 'Holding Out for a Hero' was dripping with bodies making out, grinding, dancing on their own.

The slam of the shot glasses against the sticky bar. The chanting, rising and falling, in unison, a chorus in the night. Flesh dripped. Flashes of grins and flesh imprinted on the back of my eyes. We dripped, dripped in neon. Hand-shadows on my face, on my body. Foreign hands on my flesh, familiar hands on my skin. Pearled sweat at our throats, our wrists. Eyes dribbling and drowning in pools of green and white and yellow and black. The graze of stubble. The invisible eruptions of nitrite mushroom clouds from tiny bottles. Star dust remains around nostrils like crumbling full moons.

A face in the mirror, faces in the reflection that kept staring back at me. My body slumped and sloshed. I kept turning and turning. Dancing. I danced alone. I kept dancing on my own. The press of bodies, things against me. The swell of figures and flesh. The push of faces from the shadows with grins and faces illuminated by phones so void of emotion they cannot be erased.

There were no borders there. The dark swallowed us whole. Locked the door, locked everything out, left everything behind. Hung up our skins and put on a new one. In there, I was no one. I had no past, there was no present or future. We made our offerings to the night, to the body. We were silhouettes, shadows, figures that disappeared and appeared for as long as we needed. That was the transaction. Nothing more, nothing less.

I lost myself in that club. I kept drinking and drinking. Trying to satiate a shadow in me that was always thirsty. Syrupy and golden, shots full of black potions. I gave the darkness all it craved. Dancing and stumbling and letting the shadow inside flow and leak out in my body until it sealed up my eyes without regret. Then all was dark. It was dark and dangerous, silent like a dream. I never knew where that darkness would take me. It was a game. Take the chance, roll the dice, it was freedom from me. Who will I meet, who will I become?

As I waited for a taxi with friends, a guy came up to me. He started spitting at me.

'Dirty fucking faggot.' He pressed his face against mine. 'I'm going to fucking kill you, queer.'

My friend started shouting at him. I didn't move, I didn't flinch. The alcohol stale on his breath, the rage on his face, his body tense and repulsed just by the sight of me. She pushed him away. He pulled back and carried on walking shouting homophobic slurs to the night. We hadn't done anything, simply ordered a taxi. On nights out, I've met some of my best friends, people who I'd never meet again. I've been chased down streets by heterosexual guys after heading home. Their shadows gaining on me. I kept running. I kept running. Fuelled by alcohol, fuelled by the desire to run and never stop, fuelled by letting out everything that I had bottled up. We never know who the night might spit up. It's a roll of a dice.

I navigated a world that was unfamiliar. Just another body, a story just for a night, a person that was seen as disgusting by random people on the street. The events, bars, private members' clubs, the people from backgrounds I never imagined I'd meet. I had to learn quickly how to navigate different structures, learn cultural points that I nodded along to and had to Google after. Working out how to interact with people and speak and hold myself. Making sure a country twang didn't slip out, a double negative, saying 'you was' or 'she were', sealing it all up. Having to adapt my accent and presentation to assimilate to and match my work environments or the people I was surrounded by. Searching for ways to be more interesting or impressive so I could be like them, their lives that were so unfathomable to my own. Trying to hide my uneasiness, trying to tread water in a sea that had depths I didn't know. Constantly striving to be accepted, to meet their standards but never quite meeting the requirements. Yet constantly having your identity erased because you don't quite fit their stereotype, the box that they've placed you in. Neither here nor there. Bettered yourself but not quite good enough. Fake it until you make it, play the game and you'll win. Yet never feeling like I could win, could fit in.

Numerous depictions of gay men are metropolitan, successful and wealthy. I was floating around what I had seen on TV, attending events and bars and parties with literati and successful people. While I swayed through those nights and soaked in everything around me, I never felt like I belonged. I hovered in a purgatory of 'what ifs' and 'almosts', a realm of uncertainty that they could never comprehend. Always reaching for a fruit that was just out of reach for me. Theirs wasn't a world I was used to or comfortable with. It wasn't the estate out in the countryside. I wasn't those gay men I'd seen on TV.

What impact does the 'pink pound' image that is often pushed have on people who don't belong to the middle- or upper-class? Gay men earn 11 per cent less than their heterosexual counterparts.[1] Yet we're shown to be high-flying with lots of cash to spare. Intersect this with being working class, or race, or disability, or gender – it's even more isolating and far from reality. Would I have succeeded in publishing if I had spoken like the kids on the estate? I'd spent my whole life shifting and morphing to what and who was around me to not be different. This was just another time that I had to do it, another skin to stitch together and throw on.

I've worked in places where I was called a liar about coming from a council estate. *You like opera and classical music, you love books, you write, you speak well*, were all common justifiers as to why I couldn't possibly be from an estate. As if I were using it as some privilege. Class, it sometimes seems, causes an assumption, a policing. Once it's known, you are cast into a certain box, a binary, different. Rather than judge me as a human and what I have to offer or have achieved, my background was what defined me. Other times we're seen as people to be pitied, *Well done you*, curiosities as if we are miniatures in a glass case, fascinated by this different world.

I guess my game had worked. I tricked people into believing I wasn't different and it worked. With the right words you can be anyone. Yet it didn't mask the imposter syndrome I had. The cultural reference points, the cues, the privilege, the ways of navigating. I was constantly waiting to be found out and be fired. It didn't show the amount of work I had to do to get there. But, really, it's what I've always done throughout my life, morphed and shifted, bending into what other people want and expect and need. I ran from the breadcrumb trail I was supposed to follow home and strayed from the path and into the shadows. That's what I do, I keep running. Keep running from myself, running from the words, from the story I had to follow. I felt like Icarus, waiting for the hubris to me bring me down, waiting for my wings to melt and crash back down to earth where I belonged.

After a year, I was unfortunately made redundant. I kept thinking all the work and experience would finally be enough. I sent out hundreds of applications with the result of a few interviews where I was told I didn't have enough experience or not the right experience, or would be better suited in a different department. After two years of trying to make it, I gave up. I couldn't afford to keep doing unpaid, or low paid, internships or work experience. If I hadn't had the opportunity to go home, stay with many friends sharing beds or couches, I wouldn't have been able to even attempt at working in publishing or develop my later career endeavours. But I couldn't keep pursuing something where it was clear I wasn't welcome.

Research by the Creative Industries Policy & Evidence Centre found that only 16 per cent of people working in creative industries come from working-class backgrounds.[2] When internships don't pay a living wage, are always based in London where the cost of living is so high, and entry level jobs require an insane amount of experience is there any wonder why that figure is so low? Alongside that is getting over imposter syndrome, understanding how to make it in a creative industry, nepotism, structural biases and not seeing yourself reflected in the work place or their output. There is a double disadvantage when intersected with being a woman, disabled or an ethnic minority.[3] It felt like if you didn't fit in the cookie cutter, you're not getting in.

There are very few things I have quit in my life, very few things I've been unable to overcome. I have my parents and my upbringing to thank for that – they instilled the fight and the grit in me. I was brought up on meritocracy: work hard and you'll be rewarded. I was never going to let the people who told me growing up that I'd be a nobody win. I would prove myself right. Yet this was something I couldn't beat, something structural that takes more than one person to overcome. The field was never level despite how far I climbed.

I did everything right, did everything I was taught to do. I worked hard, I studied hard, I did everything I could to put myself on a level playing field. Somehow, I had allowed myself to believe that meritocracy was a real concept. I learned quickly this wasn't the case, or that others just didn't have to work at all. It was a hard lesson to learn that no matter how hard you work, society was geared up to stop you if you are from a different background. If you are different. There is a great loss to industries that select from a small pool. A loss of perspective and training and insight and experience that is overlooked and that is reflected in both the staff and the creative output whether film, TV or books. A loss for society. I flew too high, stepped out of my place, was put back where I belonged. My wings melted and I fell and found myself, at the same time, exploring the underworld.

For a long time, I always had this drive, this hunger to destroy something inside me, to destroy myself. Or fill the void inside that kept consuming and eating and remained hungry. Smoking, binge drinking, binge eating, overexercising, not exercising, the toxic relationships. If I hurt and damaged myself enough then it would give justification and confirm what I felt inside. If I corrupt my outside, my insides, then finally I'll be what I am and have been told I am: wrong, disgusting, abnormal. A reverse Dorian Gray.

Each of us finds an outlet to channel, purge, help us through anxiety, depression, worry, shame. For some this comes through self-harm or substances or even sex. Alcohol and sex were my outlet for everything I suppressed and hated about myself. They allowed me to bury them deeper or let them out in a world where I felt shackled. They allowed me to find validity and comfort even if just fleetingly. Abuse or trauma survivors often 'use high-arousal activities of intensity, pleasure or stress and then follow with blocking strategies to balance the arousal'.[4]

I couldn't vocalise what I felt, I didn't feel like I could, like it would be taken seriously. So, I used alcohol instead to block it out or let it out in rage or emotion, releasing all the pain and hurt inside as alcohol released my inhibitions enough for it to all come out when I could no longer contain it. Crying as it all rushed to the surface. Shouting because of the hurt, because of what had been taken from me, from what had been done to me. It was a form of trying to fill the emptiness. I clutched onto acceptance. Even in the most meagre of ways. And the attention I gained, especially from a man, whether healthy or not, was a way of seeking validation, a cleansing of the shame that has been associated with my sexuality.

I'd slide under the covers alone with the afterglow of my phone to keep me company. Thinking about whether I needed to be better, upgraded for someone to like me. There were tears. I was malfunctioning. There shouldn't be cracks, no flaws. I thought I'd find validation; I'd stitch myself back together, but instead it just catalysed my sense of worthlessness.

We're sent out into the world without the proper foundation and information to protect ourselves. The fact that we leave school without a language or understanding of sex beyond the heteronormative leaves us dangerously underprepared to understand about consent, rape, assault, unwanted attention. We're not taught about intimacy, safe sex practices or healthy relationships. So many of us do not get the experience of learning about consent, boundaries and safe sex from school or as we grow up and experiment. It's thrust on us when out on the scene, apps, online, in saunas. In darkness, mute and without the language to vocalise or understand what has happened. We do not grow up learning what is acceptable and safe. We learn it on the go, through circuits of bars and clubs where we are lulled into a false sense of what is normal regarding intimacy.

SurvivorsUK reports that 45 per cent of gay and bisexual men have experienced sexual assault. Of these, 14 per cent were reported to the police.

Only 4 per cent feel in a position to seek support or tell someone.[5] Of those assaulted, 62 per cent reported the assault happened in a bar.[6] These figures, in my opinion, could be significantly higher as a direct result of lack of understanding of what constitutes sexual assault, from shame and from memory being blurred when sex and consent are affected by alcohol and drugs.

Substance use can play an integral part of being in the scene or community. Drinking and clubbing was a way for me to enter and integrate with the gay community. Before the invention of the internet, often bars, clubs and other queer venues would be the only way to meet other queer people in a safer environment and to form a community. Due to Section 28 restricting the places queer people could meet, the only places available were drinking establishments. Research shows that people feel the 'necessity of drinking in order to venture onto the gay scene and to conform to what they perceived to be community drinking norms'.[7] This can be down to a range of issues, from feeling like alcohol gives them confidence to meet other queer people to there being a lack of inclusive, alcohol-free spaces. Often, drinks will be heavily discounted for an entire night, which encourages drinking at a high-risk level where culturally there is a 'strong peer pressure to drink'.[8]

It is often cited that 'lesbians, gay men and bisexual men and women are more likely to drink alcohol, and more likely to drink excessively, than the population as a whole'.[9] There is a whole range of socio-economic and cultural factors that drive excessive drinking within the queer community, from minority stress, marginalisation, abuse, discrimination and peer pressure, through to a pervasive culture of cheap drinking. We relive our youths that we couldn't properly before, becoming Peter Pan-like, trying to reclaim and find the childhood that was taken from us.

While these spaces provide the queer community with the opportunity and space to socialise in safety, it promotes a drinking lifestyle that can lead to mental and physical health problems. Cheap alcohol, coupled with peer pressure and cultural expectations, can lead to binge drinking. Alcohol is a depressant, and can have a negative impact on mental health, making feelings of stress, anxiety and depression worse – or harder to deal with. It is possible that a dangerous cycle may form where one fuels the other, thus increasing the likelihood of mental health crises and risky drinking in the queer community.

Alongside this, drug use by the LGBT+ community is higher than the heterosexual population,[10] with gay and bisexual men three times more likely to have used drugs than their heterosexual counterparts.[11] While 6.6 per cent[12] of men who have sex with men report that they have used at least one of the three drugs associated with chemsex (GHB, mephedrone and crystal meth), and 43 per cent[13] of people partaking in chemsex have reported non-consensual sex. There is little research done into alcohol harm in the trans community and weekly unit recommendations are based on biological sex.

Throughout the queer community there is fear of accessing healthcare due to discrimination, prejudice and inadequate training and eduation for healthcare professionals around our needs. Fourteen percent of LGBT people avoid accessing treatment in fear of discrimination[14] and more than a third of trans people have avoided treatment fearing prejudice.[15] Interventions and support for substance abuse is often done through a cis, heterosexual lens meaning it very often doesn't meet our requirements. Substance support and interventions need co-designing with the community to ensure they work for us and give us the appropriate support. The social and structural restrictions and barriers impeding queer people receiving and accessing the right support, treatment and services must be removed if we are to try achieve health equity.

Some of us live with our identities, sexualities and traumas alone. This isolation and secrecy can translate into our relationships and friendships. We keep the trauma and abuse and pain buried deep without confronting, understanding or discussing it properly. It sits there from adolescence and festers until it leaks out in our adulthood. We were made to feel small, vulnerable and weak for so long that to admit something is wrong in adulthood when we are in control of ourselves is worse. It's a return to that feeling and those moments when it was out of our control and it's better to deny, hide or ignore than to regress to that feeling again. The impact society has on queer people resulting in internalised anger and shame in regards to our sexualities can result in nihilistic or self-destructive behaviour.

The shaming and othering we face in our lives directly impacts our mental health and 'another result of shame is self-destructive behaviour'.[16] I sought comfort and escape through sex and alcohol, destruction, because that was the love I felt for myself. It was the love the world had taught me I deserved. My ways of coping served as a way to block out what I was feeling as 'for the trauma survivor this means avoiding the fear and numbing the pain'.[17] Substance abuse can be a form of coping, but at its core it can be self-destruction or reconstruction to reflect what we feel deep down about ourselves or don't feel at all. It can be a way of repressing or unleashing the trauma, abuse and discrimination we have felt our whole lives. As a result of this, and minority stress, it can lead to higher levels of substance abuse in the queer community as well as catalysing existing, or drawing out, mental health problems.

The reasons behind substance use and sex are by no means applicable to all people. They can be enjoyable, healthy, recreational, relaxing, but if used in the wrong way, or purposes, can be damaging. This is not about sex or substance shaming. Sex is beautiful in all its wonderful forms and expressions and ways of enjoying it. The important part is engaging with it healthily and with consent. It's about raising awareness about the dangers that both alcohol and drugs can pose and why there is a higher prevalence of substance abuse within the queer community. It's about understanding how society can catalyse these behaviours and coping mechanisms within queer communities. We need to raise awareness not only about the risks that substance abuse can pose and the subsequent risk of assault, but its impact and catalysing of mental health conditions.

The government needs to ensure that inclusive education is provided to raise awareness from a young age about consent, assault and how to navigate the scene as an adult. We need to raise further awareness that substance abuse can lead to addictions alongside mental and physical harm. In fact, studies conducted show that having anti-homophobic interventions in schools can help reduce alcohol use.[18] We cannot keep entering adulthood blindly about sex and substances. Such support can help combat the long-term effects of minority stress and mental health problems that affect the queer community that lead to us using substances and sex as coping mechanisms. Better funded and promoted services that can help us acknowledge, address and heal from our traumas are needed.

There are increasing options in socialising in the scene where alcohol or substances are not central. There are meet-up groups that focus on activities such as hiking and climbing, book clubs, through to film groups. There are increasing alcohol-free nights as well as alcohol-free venues such as Glass House where socialising and community building are formed without the emphasis on being intoxicated. These safe spaces are vital in meeting others like us in ways that may not exacerbate pre-existing mental health problems and helping to combat them. We need to continue promoting and funding these types of initiatives.

For so long I used sex and alcohol as a way to try hide and treat my mental health issues. To forget about the pain and trauma I had experienced and was experiencing. I needed a hero. Someone to hold, someone to love, to love me in return, to make me feel validated. There have been many beds between that first bed and this one. I never thought I'd find myself flitting between rooms and lovers, trying to find me, trying to find someone to help fix the fractures inside. I didn't think I'd sink drink after drink to try forget everything that had happened.

I didn't realise the damage it was doing to me. I didn't realise the danger that it was leading me to.

Chapter Eleven

'I never want to see you hurt,' was whispered to me in the darkness. As if trying to avert a curse or the inevitable.

* * *

They always began with a hook-up, as they always seemed to do. There was never a middle to these stories. The beginning and end were wrapped up in one. I'm not sure at what point this became normal to me. The romantic who had crossed borders, flew across countries and travelled time for love. Sitting on the Tube, heading in their direction, to their promises, to their illusions. Sending the postcode to a friend, as I always did, just to be safe. Unaware that I needed saving from so much more. Jump on, jump off, mind the gap. Take the chance. The train will depart in 30 seconds. Jump on, jump off. The train was already moving, the story had begun, you took the chance, there's no getting off now. The fairy tale is beginning.

* * *

I took the chance at love, at hope. There in their arms, being pulled closer, the lips on my body. *I need you. I love you. I can't imagine being without you. Stay with me. Don't leave me. You're exactly how I imagined.* Like they had pushed me out of the crooks of their imaginations, conjured me from the recesses of their fantasies. They dripped words in my ears, a love potion that I downed. Bound to the spell they cast under sheets with snowflakes glinting on the sill, sun-baked in summer's blaze, glowing in twilight and moonshine. Unusual plot twist. This wasn't how the story was supposed to end.

* * *

Their smiles made me realise how much happiness they brought to me. A childishness long forgotten. The gifts I was bought. The hand entwined with mine leading me through galleries. Held over dinners with friends. The mornings watching each other. Whispering secrets and promises under duvets. Kissing me, another gift. *You're the one I've been waiting for.* The prince I'd been waiting for since I was a child. The one to save me, to take me away, to defend me. They promised it all and I fell for it.

* * *

A lighthouse sent its warning across the black sea, across time to warn of the sirens' call and the rocks lurking under the surface. Their calls echoing out into the darkness, the darkness in me, pulling me in like the tide. A lullaby in the night, from the past, so familiar, so dark, so dangerous. I shipwrecked myself on the rocks, sunk myself into their tides and currents, swept back up as flotsam and jetsam in tatters of lacy foam. I was salt and spray crusted and glittering in the moonlight. My hair coiled like whirlpools across my scalp. My heart in the treasure chest on the shore, waiting for them to steal it in the night.

* * *

The alcohol on our breath pulled me in and out of heady thoughts and lapses. Faces in the curves of wineglasses, lips becoming wine dark, words becoming dangerous. *Not good enough. Povvo. Fat. Not good-looking enough. Not successful enough.* Different voices, all cut the same.

* * *

The wine bottles empty, the wine glasses rimmed with red dust. I sat on the Tube, staring at the floor, trying to hide the tears that wouldn't stop.

* * *

We walked home in the still-warm night together, talking, laughing. The night buses slashing light across their faces as they gazed at me and smiled. In bed, they twined the cold amulets on my bare chest around their index fingers. Each one tugging me closer in. Wrapped around their finger. Telling me to never leave, pulling me in tightly, scared I would slip from their grip into the night. The lips on my body, their arms around me. Meshed together, bonded, grafted onto each other. It was under those hands I felt whole.

* * *

Should have worn the blue shirt. Shouldn't have trimmed my beard. Invited me over. Hasn't replied all evening. Message read, not replied. He needs me, come here. Blue tick, blue tick. 2 a.m. Not replying. Blue tick, blue tick. It was dark, it was raining. The door was locked. Message received, *It's your fault, Michael.*

* * *

They said they were sorry. It wouldn't happen again. Just a one off. They had a bad day. They needed me. Wanted me. I listened to the excuses, to the promises. I believed them.

* * *

I didn't want to be there but I was, shuttling through the night and space back to them. Something was pulling me there and I didn't know how to resist. The doors snapping open and shut. Tempting me. Jump off. Go on, I dare you. I didn't, I kept going. Swallowed in tunnels and shadow. On the same routes, routes I never thought I'd do again.

* * *

I've got to work late. I won't see them again. Busy tonight. Can't come over this weekend, I already have plans. I'm with a friend, don't worry. Nothing is happening between us. They're just a friend. They've been blocked. It's fine; I won't let it happen again. I'm busy, sorry. No plans tonight, probably just stay home. It was just the once. I can handle it. I can keep my emotions out of it. It'll just be one more time.

* * *

My phone vibrated on the table. Message received, message received, message received. Love followed by hate followed by guilt followed by blame. Repeat.

* * *

I was like a dog that came back time and time again. Scurrying, sniffling, sniffing on the ground hoping for a scrap, a crumb. Just hoping that this time I'd be given the attention, the validation, the love. I went back, of course I did. Like some dog begging, hoping to be fed some leftovers. That's how I'd been trained to be. Good boy, good dog.

* * *

The wine bottles empty, the wine glasses rimmed with red dust. I sat on the Tube, staring at the floor, trying to hide the tears that wouldn't stop.

* * *

My cousin texted saying she was worried about me. I was worried. The love that kept morphing. The darkness that kept growing. The fear that kept rising. The loneliness that kept consuming.

* * *

Fingers on my flank. Running across my skin. I didn't react, hoping that they'd get the hint when I didn't respond to those fingers creeping across my skin.
'I don't want to,' I said.
Button undone.
'Stop it,' I said.
Neck kissed.
'No.'
I stared at the walls, turning my cheek to avoid their lips. They found me. I stared at the walls because it was easier than the eyes looking at me. It was just a game for them. I gave up because I ran out of words. I didn't have the words to say what it was. I didn't have the words to understand what was happening. I gave up because that was the only way it would stop. I stared at the walls and no one said a word. No one acknowledged those two letters I said. Words have power. But only when they're listened to.

* * *

The water threaded across my body. The shower screen was steamed up with ghostly love letters appearing in the condensation. Lovers and house-mates speaking across time and memory. I tried to decipher what they wrote to each other, a love language I didn't share. I wiped away the hearts, stars and initials from the screen, wrapped my arms around my knees, rested my chin on top of them and closed my eyes. A face that wasn't my own lurked in the surface. They took it all from me. Took what was mine. I was made me a refugee from my body, my mind. The water dripping from the tap, the tears dripping into the water.

* * *

It was silent. Silence. I didn't know what to do with the silence. Without their salvos of messages. The twisting of events. The turning of words. The pull, the push. The hate. The love. It was silent, empty, like a dream. Like the magic had finally run out. Every fairy tale has an ending, just not the one that was expected.

* * *

I wasn't expecting love or affection or connection. It snuck up on me. Fell in love. Head over heels. It knocked me over, shocked me, came unexpected. Love is not an equation, it's not chemistry. We can't know when, or even why, we may connect with someone. It jumps from the lips, written on our skin, at the root of our tongues, at the tip of our fingers. We seek it out but we can never understand its origins, how to distil it, what components make it up.

It's difficult to pinpoint exactly when abuse begins. It jumps from the lips, it blooms, with every kiss, with words. It's something difficult to accept or recognise. You want to deny that it's there under the surface of the skin. It continually shifts its guise, hides behind smiles and kisses, unable to distinguish that it's happening, unable to separate it from love or affection.

It's terrifying remembering a face, only for you to recall the bizarre, fearful moment when you realised you didn't really know it at all: they were always a stranger. All those mornings cast with first light, the evenings spent memorising the way their skin shifted as their jaw clenched, the way their lips and mouth metamorphosised with worry or laughter, only for the same face to be suddenly unrecognisable. All that time looking at them and never being truly seen back. Now, in a different light, those faces I spent so long looking on was someone else's mask. The crown taken off, not a prince, but something more sinister underneath. Different faces, different words, same techniques, same abuse.

They fictionalise themselves, creating an image of your very own Prince Charming. Presenting an image that you want to see to draw you in. Romantic gestures, gifts, proclamations of love or connection, having similar interests or passions. This is often called 'love bombing', where you are made to feel you're the one they've been searching for, the one that will make you whole. Once you're in the fold, piece by piece they begin to let the mask slip.

It starts slowly. Snapping at me. Out of character. Then an insult. It was my fault; I shouldn't have said that. Then come the justifications: they were just drunk, pride was hurt, it's fine. It's followed by their regret, apologies, affection. *It won't happen again. I promise. You mean the world to me.* Repair the damage. Break it again. Break you down. Gradually over time the borders between affection and abuse blur.

At the time I didn't realise it was abusive. I knew it didn't make me feel good. I wasn't being treated well but abuse wasn't a word I would have associated with it. The twisting of words and events, the push and pull, dripping affection and following it up with an injection of hate. It took time, disentangling myself from the events and emotions, to begin to process what had happened. It took others telling me to understand. It was only when my friend told me about trauma bonding that it began to make sense.

We live, act and think in the binary. Hope and fear. Happiness and sadness. Love and hate. Fight and flight. They are a way to keep us in check, a balance to ensure that we don't live in extremes. Stasis is what keeps us functional. We oscillate between binaries, fluctuating gently and responding to the stimuli in our daily lives. They help protect us from harm, to flee when there is danger, to seek solace when we are hurt. They are fundamental for us to live our normal lives. From biology to chemistry to physics, our world is created to have neutrality and balance in order to function.

One binary so important to our normal functioning is our brain's response to safety and danger. When the two become entangled, it disrupts our normal instincts of fight/flight, what is harmful, what can save us. Trauma bonding interrupts those normal neural instincts. Trauma bonding disturbs those binaries. The binary between love and hate is shattered and your brain no longer knows how to respond in that situation and can allow you to be manipulated. It confuses you as to what is normal, what is right, what is love, what is abuse. It stops you from functioning normally and responding in a way that would keep you safe.

The person you bond to will control that binary, wielding reward and punishment and forcing it back and forth. Blurring the structures, breaking down the binaries until love and hate are merged. They belittle, devalue, distort. You're the only person in the world, they need you, depend on you. Affection, passion, attention is given via a drip that they administer. Once you've had just enough to keep you going, they'll squeeze the tube that feeds you until the point you can't take any more. Then release another dose. Reel in, devalue, discard. Reel in, devalue, discard.

They are the one, the only one, who can give it to you; the power is in their hands. You inhabit a false sense of reality where this becomes normal. Trauma bonding works on a series of belittlement and abuse followed by reward. Oxytocin is released,[1] which helps you bond to the person. When they flip and become abusive, cortisol is released thus making you seek out a protector to give you reward, which would release dopamine, this reward is associated with the abuser. It cements the bond further. It makes you seek more validation from them, more love, which in turn results in more abuse.

I didn't realise how those connections and moments were disintegrating my mental health and emotional well-being. Constantly second guessing my actions, trying to make them happy, always on edge about what mood they will be in, whether they'll hold my hand or throw some insult at me. I found myself sinking deeper into the pain and abuse I'd suppressed. I was living through the wild shifts of their emotion and behaviour: anger to love to fear to panic to passion to lust to crying. Never knowing when one would come and in which order. I began drinking and blacking out to cope, to block out what was going on. I lied to friends and family, isolated myself, kept the truth from those who truly cared for me. I became fluent in withholding the truth because I was scared of worrying others, scared of not knowing how to get out of it.

I tried to find my way back into myself again. But I had already been divided, wounds reopened that hadn't healed properly. Trauma bonding is often 'more intense when there is history of abuse'.[2] It was as if they had seen those faint scars running inside me and over time unpicked the stitches. A reverse Frankenstein where they opened them up and released the traumas of the past. What is made cannot be unmade, and they found those lingering insecurities and pain and made a new me in a body that could be controlled.

I've always felt I've had a sixth sense. I can figure someone out very quickly. Yet I didn't listen to that even when I knew they may not be healthy for me, which can be a result of shame.[3] I chose to unknow or unsee the reality of what they were like to protect myself and cover the shame. I hid away the hate and the pain and the chaos they caused behind their glamour to try lessen the hurt they inflicted. Perhaps part of me wanted to fix what I could sense was broken as I couldn't fix myself. I wanted to try protect and heal them because I couldn't do it to myself.

The abuse made me go into overdrive and try to overcompensate for the feeling of inadequacy that I felt, driven by the shame-based trauma from adolescence, and how they made me feel. Trying to be better, more impressive, better looking, better dressed, achieving more so that I could try win them over and win their affection and not the hate I was given. In the hope they'd like me more, stop the mood swings, protect myself from the hurt they were causing. I became everything: lover, friend, therapist, support. I felt like they needed me, putting more control and power in their court. The creation of a power dynamic that could be wielded due to my own feeling of insufficiency and lack of self-esteem.

Do we seek partners to create an extension of ourselves? Is the person we fall for, in love or lust, some projection of our own self? The good, the bad, the lacking. I looked for the love I thought I deserved and knew. The pain, neglect, abuse, trauma and rejection that occurs in the past, so often to queer people, can make this type of relationship feel familiar, thus mistaking it for love or affection or home.[4] Society had created an environment whereby I felt like I was nothing, worthless, shameful, not deserving of love or validation.

So, what I received came from a place where it felt right. Wrapped up in abuse, starved for validation of the person I suppressed for so long. I sought continuous validation even if it was for a moment, in the unhealthiest of ways. Being in this state where you don't feel good enough creates a power imbalance in a relationship, which 'is critical to trauma bonding'.[5] As much as we are conditioned to feel that we should be in a relationship, and love is something to strive for, we are as much conditioned to feel shame, self-hate, self-blame. We beget the love we receive.

The relationship fuelled my own need to feel validated after all the shaming, othering and discrimination I'd faced. I opened up myself to be vulnerable, to allow myself to trust in someone else, to put my hopes in someone else. I was giving myself to them, in part, as resignation of knowing that the person I truly desired would never come. There was a sense of inevitability to it all. I'd found what I felt I deserved. The previous traumas I'd been through 'may have distorted the relationship template used as an adult',[6] giving the feeling that this is what a 'normal' relationship is or what I deserved. I needed to feel love, even if it wasn't given in the needed way. I needed desire, turmoil on the outside to cover up and distract myself from the cosmic turmoil inside. You ignore the bad bits because of the hope that the original loving person you met will come back, the intermittent showers of affection will become permanent, the cycles of fear and hate will disappear.

The cyclical nature of the abuse results in you becoming increasingly powerless, becoming emotionally drained, vulnerable, subsequently becoming more reliant on them and the intermittent affection. They made me feel like I'd been made to feel previously: nothing, small, worthless. I couldn't do better. You want to leave but you can't. I repeated so many times to myself that they would never touch me again. Every time I was on my way to see them, I told myself to get off the bus. To turn around and never walk down that street again. To press the block button. I expected something instantaneous to occur, a click, a revelation that would stop myself. I couldn't. Despite the fear, the hurt, the turmoil, the pain I kept going back, kept being reeled back in. The gaslighting, the coercive control, the trauma bonding – they all merge together. Spectres of past traumas were reawakened, triggering me into that space of vulnerability.

We can only conceptualise beginning, middle and end with hindsight. During that time with them, time didn't exist. I couldn't understand where it all began and where it could ever end, or if it ever would end. If it ended, would it just be the beginning of the next one? Over a lifetime experiencing trauma, abuse, discrimination and devaluation there becomes a predisposition towards trauma-linked cues. Patterns and recognition and comfort form, which come unconsciously as 'trauma repetition is an effort by the victim to bring resolution to the traumatic memory'.[7] One abusive relationship follows another to try break the pattern, to rectify the previous one. Despite the destructive nature, it can elicit feelings of safety whereby the cyclical nature begins by finding comfort in an abuser who switches between reward and punishment. The trauma is engrained, second nature, thus doesn't feel like abuse.

Our bodies, our minds remember, even if not consciously. Trauma and abuse stay with us, it can alter the way we think, how our bodies work, how we respond to situations, how we interact with people. If not dealt with, it can be even more destructive. I felt like the years of latent and present trauma and abuse, catalysed by society's structures, which I hadn't identified or tried to resolve fostered a condition whereby I thought this kind of behaviour was acceptable. There was comfort and recognition there.

Unfortunately, society and people don't always see it this way. It's attention-seeking, they're weak, always looking for drama. *It's not as bad as it seems. He means no harm. I don't want to hear about it. Doesn't sound like anything worse than I've heard before.* These were just some of the things that were said to me when I sought advice or support. It's not physical so it's not abuse. Does it take bruises on the skin to believe? Would they believe me if they saw the bruises and cuts and torn parts inside? Because it is two men does not excuse the behaviour or lessen what it means.

The response I had was not okay and is one of the reasons why so many men don't come forward or realise themselves what they're going through. Because what we feel is denigrated and demeaned, lessened, and we are shamed for feeling that way; told to put up, shut up and get on with it, instead of seeking help and protection. It's the lack of reporting both by queer people and the mainstream media, the lack of knowledge that the abuse is happening, the shaming of not being able to admit that it has happened, the fear of not being taken seriously by the police. It can't happen because we're the same gender, we just have to 'man up'. Some are wrapped up in the conditioning that we have to be strong and protective, so many feel humiliated so don't discuss it. It makes us a lesser man. It is not just flirting or messaging or doing what boys do. It's abuse. Let this be said loud and clear: abusive relationships can happen to anyone. It doesn't matter the length of time, the gender, the sexuality, the class, the race, the age or ability. It doesn't have to be physical. It doesn't have to be romantic.

Section 76 of the Serious Crime Act 2015 created a new offence that involved coercive or controlling behaviour. In 2019/2020, 24,856 offences were reported. In 2019, only 1,112 were prosecuted, which doesn't mean they were all found guilty.[8] Divide this down by people who identify as queer – there won't be many.

Domestic abuse in the collective and legal mind is still fixed on the traditional heterosexual narrative. Legally, abuse is focused on physical and not emotional or psychological. ManKind Initiative reports that over one in three reports of domestic abuse are from men – that's over 750,000 men every year.[9] Figures vary over the prevalence of domestic abuse in the LGBT+ community. The LGBT Foundation reports that 11 per cent of LGBT people were in an abusive relationship versus 6 per cent of heterosexual women and 3 per cent of heterosexual men. Over half of the people accessing support were from GBT men.[10] A report from Stonewall in 2012 found 49 per cent of gay and bisexual men had suffered from domestic abuse.[11] A study in 2014 found that 71.7 per cent of over 850 respondents stated they had suffered at least one domestically abusive behaviour (sexual, financial, emotional or physical).[12] The figures show that abuse in the queer community is higher than in the heterosexual community, but it's not talked about. It's not supported. There are no dedicated LGBTQ+ refuge centres for domestic abuse in England. Our legal and support systems are not doing what they need to do to protect people, especially queer people, from abusive relationships.

There are still many rape myths that exist and are perpetuated, such as men can't be raped or only queer men can be raped. These narratives can stop men reporting what they've been through or mean they don't even know. The aforementioned figures could be substantially higher due to the barriers and stigma men face or the lack of education, of not knowing it had happened. Reports show 9 per cent of men have been raped or assaulted by penetration and 42 per cent experienced a sexual offence.[13] A study shows that 43 per cent of questioned men would not report to the police if they were sexually assaulted by a woman, and 23 per cent wouldn't if they were assaulted by a male.[14] The type of masculinity that is conditioned and expected creates shame and barriers for men to report or discuss these assaults; the lack of information and the myths surrounding male sexual assault is stark.

The statistics are startling. It's compounded by how our society is set up, how queer people enter into their adulthood without knowing what can happen, carrying shame and pain, a sense that we don't belong and we don't deserve any better. Heterosexual assumption, or heteronormativity, in which we are forced to live out heterosexual structures and narratives, can impact our lives in a multitude of ways whether our relationships, our sense of safety or our mental health.[15] Someone who has been particularly affected by this, or previous traumas, alongside another minority status such as race, class, disability and gender identity can give the abuser greater social status to enact the abuse, wielding the power.[16] It highlights how social inequalities and their ensuing damage on someone's mental health, self-esteem and worth can be wielded abusively.

Our society is like an abusive relationship: it gaslights us, it convinces us that what we have is what we deserve. It tells us we are accepted and equal when every day we experience cyclical trauma and discrimination from the various facets of society we interact with. It may not matter the amount of love and support we have from loved ones or family when the whole world is set up to make us feel different and less.

We carry on in life carrying this weight and pain. It's there momentarily until there is no trace that it ever existed, like a bruise. But it still lingers waiting to be exploited, drawn out by something or someone else. Our bodies are ecosystems, which, like the earth, can only sustain so much damage and repair until it starts to disintegrate and be nothing like it once was. What parts have calcified? How many neurones and nerves have been wrapped and sealed in scar tissue to stop the feeling? There is a muscle memory from trauma and abuse. Do we build immunity to love and trauma? Our bodies do so with sickness, so why not to this? My mind, my body still remembers. Even though my cells and skin and blood have regenerated. There are traces and remains that linger, a new part of my DNA. The body remembers, time is but a number.

It took time for me to leave. It took distance for me to physically remove myself to gain the clarity and perspective that something really wasn't right. I couldn't have done it without the loved ones reminding me that what I was going through wasn't healthy, the way I was being treated wasn't acceptable and that I deserved better. 'Social support is the most powerful protection against becoming overwhelmed by stress and trauma.'[17] Friends and family are essential 'to bolster the courage to tolerate, face, and process the reality of what has happened'.[18] They were the objective voices that helped me face what it was that I was going through. The reality behind the glamour, behind the words, behind the bond. They helped me sever it. It was being told about trauma bonding and coercive behaviour that helped me begin the process of understanding what had happened to me in life, how life influences and affects us negatively because of who we are, for me to start breaking the cycles of behaviour.

There is always a way out. It may take time, it may not be a switch, but there is always a route to safety. One more day, one more step, one more thought that you are better and you can do better. There is always a pathway to beginning to love yourself more, to realise that you are valid, you are strong and you deserve better than what you have.

Chapter Twelve

I'm broken. Some people say this after something difficult. Split into two, no longer the same. It's terrifying to realise that we are fragile. Despite looking whole, on the inside something has shattered. There are divisions in the self that we never realised, how someone can hurt you so much that you no longer feel complete. When severed, torn, cut away from the other half, it will never be the same entity once patched up again. What happens when life breaks up with you? Where do you go from there? How do we move on and try stitch back those pieces and recover from the past, from the trauma we've faced?

In destruction there is creation. Nothing is destroyed. It changes, forms in a new image. In the time since those relationships ended, it gave me the time to stop, think and reflect. To think about who I was, my past, how it's affected me in the present, and how I want things to be in the future. We carry an inheritance; we bring our past with us and it influences all aspects of our lives. It's one that society and structures have imposed on us, a force that shapes us into believing that we aren't good enough, we're wrong, we're different.

I thought about how many husks, iterations, versions of myself I have left behind and how many I've been forced to have in order to protect myself or survive. I was ready to shed again, leave behind the person that had ended up in such a dark and devastating situation. Sometimes we don't wish to accept it, to look back at it, to acknowledge the person we've been or the person we've been forced to become. Memories of a person gone by. It's a strange thing trying to reconcile the then and now. Nothing is truly then and done, it's a continuation. The voice of the person ten years ago while different is the same. I followed the memories of the bodies I'd been forced to live until I arrived at the most recent version: the true me.

For so much of my life, I've felt that I've had to embody someone else, a person who aligned with the expectations of others. One that society dictated I had to be like: masculine, straight, working class, gay, middle class. It got to the point where I no longer belonged in my own body, couldn't be who I truly wanted to be. So many narratives are set up by society for us to tightrope along. We're forced into chapters that we don't belong in. We feel like we're not one of the cast if we don't play along with the role we've been given by life. I was haunted by the ghosts of all these other people I've been, the faces of the past, the whispering of the trauma and the abuse and the pain under the surface that I didn't want to listen to.

It would have been easy to repeat my behaviour and patterns that I'd consistently followed throughout life: erase the memories, push them down and away. Forget them rather than live with them. Be haunted by the spectres of them when I least wanted it. But this was a reckoning point. I couldn't keep moving through life without trying to understand the events of my life, how society had shaped it, how I ended up believing being abused was what I deserved. People say you'll forget, you'll get over it. Things aren't forgotten, they lie dormant, entwined with nerves and RNA. They'll rekindle unexpectedly, shape you unknowingly. We cannot forget or ignore. We cannot cut out the rot and think the fruit is still good. The good and bad need to coexist in order to move on.

Leaving the abuse behind was like a full stop in my life. A death followed by life. It allowed me to stop, momentarily, before allowing me to start again. A new beginning, a new opportunity to evolve. It was whether that evolution was towards further chaos or not. I could let this moment consume me and continue to wreak further chaos to my mental health, my friendships and my future relationships. Or I could try to change for the better. Use it as my moment to understand who I was, why things had happened, to see me in my entirety. Unleash the chaos inside, cut the bindings of my existence to create a new me, a me in my own image. Nothing dies, it just changes. Full stop.

I'd spent the majority of my life using a series of distraction techniques to avoid dealing with what I'd been through. Exercise, partying, alcohol, work, running to events, writing, suppressing, had all been used so I could try and run from the shame, the fear, the pain I'd carried throughout life without realising how it was changing me from the inside out. It meant I didn't have to confront the fractures within me. I didn't have to speak about it, just carry on, be okay, as that's what we're taught to do. Be silent, not complain, be grateful for our lot. It meant I didn't realise how society was geared up to continuously gaslight queer people to the point where we break, feel broken, don't believe that we have the right to be safe and happy and equal from the very point we are born.

Words have power to hurt. They also have the power to heal what has been broken. I'm beginning and trying to learn to speak up more. For a long time, I felt I had to carry everything by myself, bottle it up, internalise it and keep going on. Hiding my problems, fears and anxieties doesn't make them go away. Voicing them doesn't make me weak. Not just for myself, but in case there is someone else out there who is feeling the same and alone, for someone else who may not have realised – like I did – what they have gone through. Hearing a story similar to yours can be transformational.

We need support at times. We're not burdens. I always felt like I would worry or scare or upset someone by telling them what was going on or how I was feeling. Telling part-truths or nothing at all. We give and we take in our support systems and it's important to do both. I'm starting to break away from that boyhood conditioning to bottle it up, not speak up and out, not to feel emotional. It has done too much damage, it does too much damage. We cannot progress as people if we don't speak our truths. Words can heal.

In the steps to recovery, 'it is critical to communicate with loved ones close and far'.[1] Not only to let them know how we are feeling, what we have gone through or are going through, but taking the step in '(re)connecting with our fellow human beings'.[2] This is vital for us to know that we have support and love in the face of the pain, trauma or abuse we've gone through. This is to reinforce that not every person is out there to make us feel small or different. Trauma bonds are powerful in that they isolate us from the people who provide a network of safety and true love. Our 'attachment bonds are our greatest protection against threat',[3] and 'study after study shows that having a good support network constitutes the single most powerful protection against becoming traumatized'.[4]

Our loved ones are so often one of the most essential components in recovering from trauma, abuse or mental health problems. There are many who cannot rely on family for love, support and understanding. So many queer people are rejected by the very people who should love them unconditionally, or feel they cannot go to them out of fear or lack of understanding. There is no hope or escape. There is not the right support from loved ones or carers or from society.

That's why so many of us have friends so close that they are our chosen family, often the ones we go to first, the ones who know everything. I know my luck and privilege that I have love and support from my family and chosen family. It wasn't just receiving that initial support when coming out to everyone that helped me to begin to accept and love who I was. It was the continued love and support as I dealt with the issues I've gone through, the painful acknowledgement of the trauma I've been through and how it has altered me, getting me through and out of the abuse. They were the lights that guided me through the darkness, the stars at night that helped me remember that there is always another day, another chance of hope. The ones who always had their arms and hearts open when I needed it even when I didn't think I did or could.

I've been lucky, so lucky. Life has thrown some tough things at me, others have it much worse. I've picked myself up and my family and friends more often than not have carried me literally and figuratively. They've held me as I cried, they waited until I could breathe again, through the tears and the sobs and the choking on the phone; they listened to me drunk-ramble and shout and rage to try rid of myself of the hate and anger and pain that

I buried so deep inside me. They've taken me out and we've danced and laughed and held our stomachs from the laughter cramps. We've curled up on couches and beds, sat and talked, listened to anxieties, said nothing at all but made sure they were a presence next to me.

They've supported every step, every misstep and made sure I got back on the path when I was ready, sometimes pushing me into it to make sure I kept going, that I became the person they saw, not the one I thought I was. I know I've driven you crazy at times. I hope you all know how grateful I am. This is a love note for all of you, each one of you that has helped me get over the hurdles, who has shown undying love and loyalty and patience. I wouldn't be here without you in all senses of that meaning. You keep reinforcing in me that life is good and I'm worth something more than I've been made to feel. You're the ones I live for and the moments we spend together. You have accepted and loved me unconditionally. I couldn't have made it through these times without you. Without you, I could have quite easily given up.

Without you, I couldn't have pulled myself out from those relationships. From the darkness that kept pulling me deeper. You're the ones who kept reminding me that it wasn't right, I had to leave, I deserved better, it wasn't love, I'm better than them, I didn't deserve to be treated that way, when I couldn't convince myself of those things. 'Being truly heard and seen by the people around us, feeling that we are held in someone else's mind and heart,'[5] can be the biggest thing in leaving or staying in an abusive relationship, in trying to move past mental health issues. Having someone there to listen, tell you that something isn't right and help you through it can make all the difference.

You've fought for me, physically and verbally, defended me, protected me from the world, from people, from myself. You've been my voice when I didn't feel I had one. You allowed me to believe, to believe in myself, that I deserved better, to believe that the world can be better. You never saw me or treated me as different like the world did. I've followed the bread trail you left for me, and it hasn't always been an easy path, but what got me to the end is you and knowing you're waiting for me there. I've always been stuck in a fairy tale book, hoping that one day a prince, a hero, would come and save me. You are the heroes.

I began to learn to put up boundaries instead of walls. Learning and implementing what I will and won't accept from others and myself. Not just to protect but to grow. Surrounding myself with people who will support and champion me to be the best person and for me to give that in return. Treasuring and nurturing those healthy relationships are so vital in order to foster a healthy relationship with yourself and others.

I destroyed love because I couldn't find it for myself. I accepted destructive love because that's what society taught me I deserved. I repeated patterns of rejection and destruction as that was what felt normal. I always wanted to be more than I was because I didn't feel I was enough. It's only now that I realise that I am. I'm more than enough. I spent so much of my life feeling like who I was wasn't valid. I needed to stop finding acceptance and validation from others and accept myself. I needed to stop apologising for who I am. I needed to stop trying to keep others, the world happy, and in turn sacrificing my own happiness. I needed to consider the ways that I didn't love myself in order to start doing that. There were many and there were many that were difficult to confront and accept.

There was always the fear of: who is going to love me? First, myself. It's never too late to learn love, especially for yourself. I had to take the time to fully accept and love myself. Aristophanes stated that when humans were split in two at the beginning of the world, we were in continuous pursuit of our other half. I always thought this would be a partner but I've learned that it was myself. I had to find myself, bring together those fragments inside and stitch them together. Like the Japanese art, *kintsugi*, that uses golden lacquer to fix ceramics, I coiled myself in gold to piece the parts together again. Embracing the flaws, accepting the past to find the beauty in the differences that I'd been told had none.

The media rolls out for their annual coverage of Pride to broadcast the smiling sun-drenched faces and glittered bodies that scatter rainbows across the streets basking in their perceived equality. We're shown to the world as perpetually happy, forever young, a community that has no fear. The world has come so far, we have come so far, our fight is over, equal rights for all. We're given our one moment to shine and for the world to feel reassured all is okay for the queer community. A glamour, just a deception to hide the pain underneath those beaming faces. We live in an illusion.

Yes, our rights are the best they have ever been. Yes, our representation and visibility are better than before. Our ability to connect is easier, our acceptance is generally better. But our society is still fundamentally flawed. We cannot continue to be grateful for what we've been given when so many facets of our society result in long-lasting damage, when our rights are now being reversed across the world and queerphobic attacks are increasing. We are not broken; we don't need to be fixed. It's society that needs fixing.

We go through life carrying this inheritance, a burden, a guilt without understanding that it is not us, it is society that slowly conditions us into this state of being. I'd leaned into society's deception that everything was okay when year by year something inside was disintegrating, my mental health was crumbling, my self-esteem was so low that I was careering into abuse without knowing it. We seek validity of who we are. When that validity is rejected throughout our lives, we become disassociated from our identities, feeling like we don't belong in our bodies or society, deep-rooting shame for who and what we are throughout our lives when we should be feeling safe and comfortable and loved.

I've lived with those different identities competing inside of me, fighting for superiority over which belonged most, which was the worst, all cowering from the spectre of shame that lined my body. All the while society beat them all into submission. Stay in your lane, don't rise above your station, know your worth. How could I be working class *and* gay? How could I be gay *and* masculine? How could I be working class *and* feminine? None of these plots followed the one society had given me. I decided that I couldn't unmake myself anymore, but threaded together all parts of my identity to renew and strengthen my identity.

My questions of what it means to be a gay man from a council estate who didn't live up to the heterosexual masculine ideal no longer mattered. The realisation was that the policing of my identities was the issue, not my identities. The feeling of othering, of difference, will still lurk there but I needed to understand where it came from in order to move forward. I reached out to the community more, whereas previously I'd been scared to embrace it.

I spoke to other queer people, understanding their lives and experiences, what their journeys were.

I started reading and studying queer history and lives to understand what had happened to our ancestors and how we reached the point we are at now. Reading about the spectrum of gender and sexuality, the strength of working-class people, many of whom were people of colour and trans, who had the strength and will and belief that we deserved a place at the table and fought for our equal rights. I read up on law and psychology and sociology and trauma and abuse. I read about the injustices put on minorities, how structures are set up to keep us down, how they have been broken down. I learned how the past and present influence us, and where we need to go to fight for our rights and what needs to happen in society for us to live in a safer world where it doesn't condition us to think of difference as inherently wrong or abhorrent, but celebrates our individualities. Difference isn't bad, it's powerful, it's beautiful. History and the past are there for us to learn from, to grow, to stop cycles.

I began to understand how we connect, how our feelings are the same, interconnected, different, similar. I saw reflections of my own story, people who had realised that they'd been through relationships or experiences that they hadn't known were unhealthy. Society and people had made them feel different, had had the same impact on their mental health, the feeling of shame. This is the importance of vocalising our stories, our struggles, our truths. Sharing can get us through so much, it's what makes us human, it's how we evolve. We are all part a wider narrative that society inflicts on us. I began to feel less alone in who I am and what I've gone through. Society, its systems and structures, subject many of us to the same fate. This is shared.

'Trauma is not stored as a narrative with an orderly beginning, middle, and end.'[6] This played a fundamental role in my healing. It helped me understand that the abuse I experienced wasn't an isolated product, my mental health problems weren't an isolated product. They weren't neatly tied up in a beginning, middle, end. Trauma will surface at many points in life, not just at the trauma's conception, and can influence you in a multitude of ways. Just because it may not have an obvious impact at the time doesn't mean it hasn't affected you inside, hasn't altered how you react to the world, to yourself, others around you. The body records everything, it changes even if nothing looks like it has changed; nothing is destroyed even if it may be forgotten. Trauma doesn't just appear and disappear. We get up every day shouldering a weight even if we can't feel it. The everyday microaggressions, the long-standing abuse and othering from childhood, the shame, the guilt. It shifts and influences; blooms and explodes in ways we can't predict. It hovers over us, waking up and not knowing why we feel down, what's wrong, why we don't feel like carrying on, why we're so tired. Humans are resilient, we can function for years, decades, until the body or mind finally signal that it can't handle it anymore. Our mental health can only take so much.

Healing is not a switch. It's one step at a time, sometimes steps backwards or sideways. I've tried antidepressants, been through therapy, written and written to understand, read, thrown myself into different activities that would help me feel better in myself. There is not a magic trick to overcome what we've been through and go through. No potion to drink that'll erase the past and transform us into an entirely different person. We don't live in fairy tales. My journey out of abuse, my path to begin to deal with my mental health issues will not be the same for everyone. The biggest part was to live my life, live who I am and who I want to be. Embracing and loving my truth. Not what others, not what society expect of me. See myself in all its entirety, its beauty, its importance. If there is one thing to remember, it is you are beautiful and you are valued. We cannot let the world minimise us.

That journey still continues. There is no failure. It's a series of falling on and off the band wagon, it's a process that will continue. But there is a route for everyone. That is why we must continue to talk, to heal together, to speak up, to challenge. The world is full of systemic barriers and structures that are in place to bring us down, to make us feel different, to weaken us. We cannot change the world if the world doesn't understand the realities that we face, how our lives are affected by what has been set up around us. We cannot change the world by doing it by ourselves or taking each other down. We have to dissect what is going on around us in order to understand what it is we need to do to make that future better.

We have to understand the past, how it affects our present and how we can shape the present into a different future. They don't work in isolation. We all have many beginnings and many endings, it's at what point we start to define ourselves. Finding that point is key to beginning to address and work through the trauma. Continuing to find those new beginnings, finding those ending points to move on and start a new chapter in our healing. We take our history with us. We cannot destroy the past. We cannot change it. We can evolve from it though. We can learn from it, accept it and move forward as a different person. *Ad lucem*, towards the light, was embroidered on the red badge I wore on my blazer at school years ago. Another day, another dawn, one more step towards the light.

Epilogue

The light dripped, spun sugar, from the leaves and branches. The dog snuf-
fled around in the ferns, seeking out something hidden, memories and
shadows, in the greening undergrowth. The dew outlining footprints in
trodden-down grass. My footprints that I was retracing from yesterday, the
same route I'd been taking the last few weeks. I was retracing routes and
footprints from the past, ones I'd made for years.

The world was silent, it had stopped. I'd stepped back in time and time
was broken. I was back on the estate, having moved home during the pandemic. Going back to the woods where I grew up for my daily walk. It was
empty. The voices and faces from my childhood gone, kids no longer played
there. Their ghosts, my ghosts, still played in the shadows, in the rustle of
the breeze through leaves and snowdrop bells. Whispers of our past selves
still trying to find the edge of the woods.

To get back home you can walk through the old estate, now redeveloped
with young couples, families and commuters. The community, the togeth-
erness, the networks had gone. The old alleys and houses and paths gone.
Different streets and people, the history unknown to them, my history now
just an echo of our childhood selves calling down the allies. A lost lullaby.
It felt so small, so distant from the boy that once wandered those streets. A
place that changed me so much now just a bunch of buildings that I walked

through to get to the woods. It was different and so was I. The kid who grew up there had gone on to achieve more than he ever possibly could have imagined, what others could have imagined.

As I wrote in my room, the windows open, I heard kids out on the park. One was telling another how his cousin is lesbian and has a girlfriend, the other replied, 'Cool.' It was the same park I had played on, throwing myself from the swing at the top of its trajectory, sprinting across to get home in time for tea, running from the words that I was branded with. Over twenty years had passed, there were still kids playing on the same green, but they were different. A new generation where being queer isn't different, it's not wrong.

This is not to say that prejudice and discrimination don't exist, they do, but attitudes *are* changing. That never would have happened when I was in their shoes. At my desk, I cried for the child me who didn't have that experience. I cried because there was hope. Hope that kids would grow up without fear of who they are, without the shame, without being made to feel their difference was wrong. They could leave childhood with pride, enter their adulthood with confidence and hopefully avoid some of the injustices and pain that society made many of us feel.

Writing most of this book on the estate was a surreal experience. In my childhood room, in the silence, in the world's silence I finally stopped. I was silent and still and I moved through time and space and lives. I listened to that little boy practising dance routines to Britney. The little boy who pulled himself up on the chin-up bar thousands of times, the marks on the door frame still visible under new layers of paint. I listened to the teenage me who felt he had to bury his true self behind muscle and sinew. The marks of adolescence still in my mind, still visible under years of history. I pushed myself through memories and into the skins I'd lived and the skins I no longer wanted to live. I wrapped the ghosts around me, I embraced them and listened to them. Stayed silent and let them tell me their stories, the events they lived and the words they had heard and been told.

I peeled back the layers and the scars and the love and the pain and the forgotten things that weren't allowed to surface to find that person who had been lost, the child that wasn't allowed to breathe, the me that society had never allowed to dance out into the world and past the borders of the woods. There in that room, while the world seemed to be falling apart, I wrote to try put myself back together. I'd stopped running, been forced to stop, and it gave me the chance to say hello, to hold the person I'd be running from. Nothing is destroyed, it just changes. Reliving the time I had there, both the pain and incredible experiences, I began to understand how it influenced my sexuality and gender but also my resolve, resilience and creativity.

Being back there allowed me to analyse my childhood with a different lens. To reclaim a love for the council estate and all that it gave me. To be proud of that little estate and the person it made me into. No one else will have a childhood like it and I'm grateful that I didn't come out like a cookie-cut person. It helped me look at the rest of my life with a fresh lens too. It was a strange turn of events that of all places in the world, it was on the estate that I was offered representation by my agent. After that call, I came downstairs and sat on the back doorstep and sobbed into my hands. My mum came in and I told her about the offer.

'Why are you crying for? It's what you've always wanted!' she said as she held me.

'I just never thought it could happen.'

I cried for that little boy on the estate where so many people made him feel different and wrong, who was told he'd be a nobody. I'd done it for him and for all the other kids who were told they were different. Really, there was no other place I should have been told other than on the estate. It's what made me, it forged my love of books and writing. It forged me. It's only with time, reflection, growth that I've learned that difference is not wrong.

Being made to feel different can be destructive, it can be traumatising. Difference is just as powerful. Difference is what made me. I lived through my life resenting that I'd been made to feel that way, to feel that I don't belong in the world or even in my own body, consumed by the pain and trauma that it had caused. The world we live in conditions us, pressurises us into homogeny. Bashing and forcing us into submission so we are just like everyone else, living in the same narrative. We should not be eradicating difference; we should be celebrating it. It's what makes our world, humanity, so powerful and beautiful. Difference is what gives us culture, it's what gives us expression, it's what give us hope. Without wanting to make a difference, things can't change.

Not fitting into the narrative is what allows us to disrupt it, to see its flaws, to see how it can be improved. Society and people will find a way to make us feel small because of who we are and our difference. It is making ourselves big and taking up the space they say we don't deserve that has gotten us this far in our fight for equal rights and our position in society. It is easy to be silent, it's even easier for us to be silenced by the world and its structures that have been constructed over centuries to make us feel that we don't have a voice or a place at the table.

There were so many moments when writing this book when I thought to myself that I should stop and it's not worth it. It would be easier to keep silent. But that's what the world wants: to feel like my voice isn't powerful, my story isn't worthy, my words aren't important. Our lives and our voices and our narratives matter. We do have a place at the table and it's our belief in who we are that has kept us there, to keep talking, to keep fighting.

There are many paths and narratives in life and so often it feels that we don't have a choice in the one that's given to us. We do. Every single day we get up, we are brave. Every day we get up and choose to live and love and fight is an act of resistance. We are so strong to take on a world that makes us feel that we shouldn't be in it. Every step we take, every day we keep going, we are changing that narrative, we are making our own paths by not allowing the world to win. We create who we are, products of our own narratives and the ones given to us. We need to choose our terms just as we have always done. We have created our own culture, evolved from our history, forced our way into the world with light and love and resilience and power to tell the world, 'Fuck you.'

We are our own protagonists and we cannot stop the fight and allow the world to convince us that we don't deserve more or better. To be lulled into a false sense of security that things are fine, our work is done or there is nothing we can do at all. Society gives us an inheritance that shapes us, pressurises us, changes us. It's a narrative we don't ask for, often we don't belong in, or deserve to be in. We spend most of our lives trying to unlearn that conformity. After not seeing a university friend for a while, she said

that I seemed 'more gay'. It was a result of years of unpicking that heterosexual narrative and beginning to love and embrace who I am, to reject the
conformity and begin to live the true me.

In turn, we have our own inheritance from our ancestors who sacrificed
and fought for us to get to the position we are in now. We need to continue
their legacy and continue to fight and protest and change the inheritance
the next generation of queer people pick up.

Difference is born on the lips, but it is society that shapes those words and
actions. The mental health issues we live with, the abuse we go through,
the stigma, prejudice and discrimination we face do not exist in a vacuum.
They are created and catalysed in our societies. Born in structures, institutions, policies, traditions and ignorance. Governments, people, the media
treat our lives and existence as a debate, a game. We are used as scapegoats,
targets in political games and tactics, as shown by anti-queer policies
implemented by governments. From the Trump administration, the 'Don't
Say Gay, Don't Say Trans' bill in Florida passed in March 2022, there are over
200 similar proposed bills across the States, similar legislation passed in
2021 in Hungary and the 'no queer zones' in Poland.

Organisations are rescinding their support of Stonewall's diversity
programmes, many as a direct result of anti-trans rhetoric. The same techniques that were used against gay and lesbian people in the 1980s are now
being used against our trans siblings. Our position in society is as perilous
as ever. Rights can be given. They can as easily be taken away. Time goes
backwards, a series of beginnings and endings colliding.

The world thinks that now we can get married the job is done. It is clear
this is not the case. Over the past six years, homophobic hate crimes rose
210 per cent and transphobic hate crimes rose 332 per cent.[1] Discrimination,
murder, bullying, prejudice, mental health crises, trauma, institutionalised
queerphobia, where hate crimes are ignored or not handled properly by the
police through to anti-queer law and injustices still exist in our society.

Research done by Drinkaware revealed that the pandemic lockdowns
affected the mental health of the queer community more than the population as a whole and were more likely to drink once lockdown ended.[2] The
LGBT Foundation reported that during the first coronavirus lockdown

from March to May 2020, they received 25 per cent more calls about suicidal thoughts, 65 per cent more about domestic violence and 50 per cent about substance abuse.[3] Many queer people were trapped in situations and homes that were dangerous, oppressive and restrictive. They were away from safe spaces, their own spaces, and isolated from normal support networks, highlighting how important our safe spaces and networks are. The pandemic has further highlighted the structural inequalities and the impact this has on queer mental health. More so than the heterosexual population – there is a clear reason for this. We still don't inhabit a world that is safe and fair.

The mental health of the queer community has for too long been ignored and swept under the carpet. Same-gender abuse has barely even reached the surface. The numerous statistics mentioned in this book regarding queer health and abuse, and how the toxic pressures and conditioning around masculinity is one of the reasons why suicide is the biggest killer of young men, shows that we need to act, talk and change our society, laws and education systems. Society has created conditions whereby the combination of gender and queerness can create a potent and dangerous intersectionality. We cannot let the clock be turned back.

Violence is cyclical. We find it in childhood. The violence against our gender expression, verbal and physical. The violence against our sexuality, verbal and physical. The violence against our difference, verbal and physical. It carries into our adulthood where we perpetuate this violence we endured as children on ourselves, our relationships, to others. We have to break the cycle.

So many things that happen to queer people are often accepted, normalised and not confronted, not met with resistance, no regret, resignation. Whether this is out of fear, not knowing what has happened or the way society is set up to stop us understanding or from the media and governments ignoring the effects society, policy and culture have on queer people. We navigate a world that likes to gaslight us. Society reflects the abuse I went through: it makes us feel like we're safe yet chips away at us until we give up, takes our voice away and makes us feel like we don't deserve better.

The phrase from the 1980s 'Silence = Death', created by a collective in New York City to raise awareness and support during the AIDS crisis, rings as true now as it did then with our rights under attack, our bodies under attack, our mental health under attack. We are shackled by conditioning, law, education, society, people. So many of our stories will be ignored by history, swallowed into silence purely because of our gender and sexuality. Words can inflict difference, shame and hate, but they're also key in reclaiming power over our lives. Our stories and lives have been gagged; society has neglected to equip us with the tools we need in life. We cannot become silent. We have to begin to learn to speak up and out. It can be fatal if we're coerced into believing or accepting that we don't have a voice or that this is our lot. Our job every day is to believe there is worth in who we are. Pick ourselves up and keep fighting. Every day is a fight. Every day we get to choose who are and what we will do.

I could have stayed quiet about my story. Swept it into the closet and not thought it had any significance. It's better to forget, nothing really happened at all. Writing: it's invasive. You have to cut yourself open and dig deep inside. In my writing I tried to make sense of myself, of the pain in the world, the trauma of my life. It is not the book I ever expected to write, events I never expected to ever happen to me. But it is one that is needed.

My journey is not everyone's journey. My experiences are my experiences. I recognise I am a white, cis man. I am not trying to homogenise queer people and group experiences as essentialist or collective. There are so many other intersections and backgrounds that influence each life and impact them in a different way that need to be explored. Mental health and abusive relationships are unique to every person and don't necessarily relate to sexuality or gender. They find their roots in many places. Indeed, they will not happen to every person. There may be events in this book that are similar to yours, it doesn't mean it will happen to everyone. Going through abuse or trauma or discrimination does not mean you will end up in an unhealthy relationship. Nor are the reasons I explore behind the crisis exhaustive, there are so many more that need to be explored and discussed. Not every one of you will recognise what I have explored as your truth or agree that they contribute to mental health problems or facilitate abuse – that is your right and that is your journey.

This was mine to try to understand what happened to me. I draw on my own life and apply this to what I see in society and the systemic issues that pervade our society and how this can apply to us, our friends and loved ones. This is one experience and shows that there this so much more that needs to be explored in our community alongside other intersections, lives and voices. To expose what society does to us, to start conversations, to reveal the injustices, to uncover the unreported and unspoken abuses and pain that happen in the queer community. It's about beginning conversations.

Writing for me has always been about necessity and survival throughout my life. Even when it wasn't to work out something in my mind, it was creating a different world, a new world. Writing this book has been out of necessity and survival for my past self and my present self but more importantly my future self and for your future self. My story and journey can only be my own. It was important for me to begin a conversation, an attempt to expose what it is in our society that creates these conditions where we feel alone, our mental health suffers, abusive relationships go unspoken about or unknown, and we feel like there is no hope in the world. It was important to assert that the way we feel isn't a personal failure but because of how society is built and how it forces us to be. It was important to try and figure out ways to overcome those issues. Not everyone will hold governments or organisations accountable at the highest of courts, or found charities to support queer people. Everyone has a voice and we all need to use them.

Section 28 was revoked in 2003; in 2005 same-sex civil partnerships were legalised and same-sex marriage became law 2015. In 2019, 86 per cent of the population in the UK agreed that homosexuality should be accepted by society, compared to 75 per cent who said that homosexual activity was 'always or mostly wrong' in the 1980s. Male rape became recognised in law in 1994 and the 2003 legislation made victims of rape gender neutral. The Domestic Violence, Crime and Victims Act 2004 allowed same-gender couples the same entitlement and protections as heterosexual couples. LGBTQ+ people have never had so many rights or so much representation in history – yet same-gender abuse and mental health problems are rife within the community. Clearly there are systemic failures embedded in our culture, beyond what legal ratifications have resolved. That needs addressing. We have come so far in our civil rights movement, yet the fight is still not over. We need to keep vocalising for change and awareness to stop these issues.

Our progress cannot solely be from a legislative stand-point. It is not the only thing that enacts change in our society. From before someone is born, we need to shift our mindset how we approach that child. To shift away from heterosexual assumption, gender binary and heterosexual narratives, expectations and boxes that enclose a child in a life that is defined by their assigned sex and assumed heterosexuality. Our schools need to reinforce this in how they approach subjects, sex and well-being education to ensure that our students go through school knowing there are others like them, it is normal, and how to enter adulthood fully prepared to enter a relationship or have sex. Our industries need to be better at having inclusive representation to ensure inclusive and positive representations of queer people with all their intersections. It affects not only our own self-images but those seen by the wider public, too.

We need to come together as a community more. Activism is better as a collective, a force that can't be stopped. We cannot be divided in ourselves; the world is already trying to do that. It was all the community coming together that allowed us to have the rights that we have now. If we see another person struggling, reach out to them – the people around us can literally save lives. We need to talk about our experiences and lives more with each other. I didn't know others had gone through similar things to me, and speaking with them about my experiences they also realised or opened up that they had similar ones, too. It normalises and explores our issues, we're not alone, it allows us to open up and understand what we've gone through and how to tackle it together. We can find a commonality in our experiences and start breaking down the shame and the traumas.

On an individual level, we need to look after ourselves. Surround ourselves with people who care for and support us, find spaces where we are accepted. We need to recognise that mental health is a real threat. We are not a burden for asking for help or support from loved ones. Nor are we a burden for asking for support from our healthcare systems. There are many support lines and services that are dedicated to queer people that can give you guidance and advice when you feel you can't reach out to other people. It can be easy to bear the weight of our anxieties, abuse, worries and trauma on our own because for some of us that has always been the way. It doesn't have to be. The biggest task can be asking for the support.

You are enough. Even though so many times it feels we have to try harder, be smarter, stronger, just to be on the same field. You are enough. You have so much life, you have so much beauty, don't hide yourself away. Stop trying to fit in, because we don't and that's our strength. Our difference is our power, it's our right, it's ours. Certainty is not a gift for us. We can make a certainty just like our ancestors believed when they ensured legislation was changed, protections were put in place.

Our world is changing and so much for the better. Our visibility and representation are so much better; in general, the public is so much more accepting. When the world told me I was alone, I went out and found a world that was loving and accepting. I found a community that was big and wonderful and queer and kind. Our community is special. We need to come closer together, talk more, to protect ourselves and not isolate. Many people before us couldn't be out openly, and many still can't, but we have more ways of connecting and finding each other now. We deserve to live in a world without shackles or gags, where our potential is unlimited. We shouldn't have to overcome obstacles in order to feel like we deserve love. We deserve a life of being told you'll get true love, your love matters, of seeing healthy reflections of our culture and lives.

While this book is very much a gay story, it's also unfortunately one defined by a heterosexual narrative, heterosexual structures, a heterosexual world. Our allies are so important. This is not just a responsibility, a problem, a battle that queer people should or have to face alone. It is every person's duty to take responsibility and change, disrupt and fight the narrative and society that fosters these conditions. Each one of us has a duty for the narratives that are supported and disseminated. As much as this is a book to help queer people understand the issues we face, why things happen to us, it is one for cis-heterosexual people to realise how the world impacts others beyond the heteronormative. We cannot do this fight alone. It is for all of us to pull down those bars that constrict us.

Life has seemed to be a series of breaking and rebuilding. This is what we need to continue to do to get us to where we need to be in society. Break down the barriers that hold us back, build up the structures that can support us. Tear off the gags that have kept us silent for so long. To start conversations, to tell our lives and stories. To call out what is wrong and what is right. To no longer be silent, but to scream, shout and sing our stories. To realise that each and every one of us has a voice that is important and valid and strong.

For so long, I didn't believe who I was or that my story was valid or important. I buried it and let the pain and hurt affect me from the inside out. There are many beginnings and endings. This one is ending but maybe, hopefully, it'll be the beginning of something else. Now it's your turn, to speak your truth. Difference is born on the lips: it's our time to make a difference.

Support Services

Galop
www.galop.org.uk
0207 704 2030

The National 24 Domestic Violence Helpline
0808 2000 247

Survivors UK
www.survivorsuk.org/
020 3322 1860

The LGBT Foundation Helpline
https://lgbt.foundation/
0845 330 3030

ManKind
www.mankind.org.uk/
01823 334244

MindOut
https://mindout.org.uk/
01273 234839

Mind
www.mind.org.uk/

Samaritans
116 123

CALM
0800 58 58 58

Thank You To

My family. You gave me love, you gave me support, you gave me protection, you gave me the world. You made me fearless, you made me believe I could be, and achieve, anything I wanted. You made me me. I will be forever grateful for your unconditional love, support, understanding and sacrifice and to call you my family.

My nan, you brought so much light to the world when it often seemed so dark.

Steph – my twin – a thank you could never do justice to or embody how much you mean to me. I wouldn't be here today without you. I wouldn't be the person I am without you. There are thousands of words I could write, but none sum it up more than: I love you.

Fran, it's been over twenty years and I still count my blessings that we ended up in the same tutor group. All the laughing, dancing, adventures, support, championing, picking me up, editing, bed sharing, friendship, love, screaming – you're the best friend anyone could ask for.

Jenny, for giving me the power to understand what I was going through, for giving me the ability to break away and to recover. For your friendship, the walks, the support, the chats, all the workshops and the edits. This book wouldn't exist without you.

Anna and Una, my musketeers, my muses, my sisters.

All my friends for the love, the support, the adventures – the best bunch I could ever ask for.

Abi, Callen and Jo for believing in the power of this story and for making it a reality. For championing and fighting and supporting a voice that has been long ignored. For understanding the importance of it for so many people.

James, for the use of your beautiful image on the cover design.

The whole team at Flint Books who made this book what it is.

The Society of Authors for the financial support received from the Authors' Foundation.

Notes

Prologue

1   HRC Foundation, 'Sexual Assault and the LGBTQ Community', Human Rights Campaign, accessed 1 April 2022, www.hrc.org/ resources/sexual-assault-and-the-lgbt-community

2   April Guasp and James Taylor, 'Domestic Abuse: Stonewall Health Briefing', Stonewall, January 2015, www.stonewall.org.uk/system/ files/Domestic_Abuse_Stonewall_Health_Briefing_2012_.pdf

3   Chaka L. Bachmann and Becca Gooch, 'LGBT in Britain: Health Report', Stonewall, 2018, www.stonewall.org.uk/system/files/lgbt_in_ britain_health.pdf

4   José Esteban Muñoz, *Cruising Utopia: The Then and There of Queer Futurity* (New York City: New York University Press, 2009), p.65.

5   Gavin Brown, 'Listening to Queer Maps of the City: Gay Men's Narratives of Pleasure and Danger in London's East End', *Oral History: Pleasure and Danger in the City* 29, No. 1 (Spring 2001), 48–61.

Chapter Two

1   Michael Schwalbe, 'Identity Stakes, Manhood Acts, and the Dynamics of Accountability' in Norman K. Denzin (ed), *Studies in Symbolic Interaction* (New York: Elsevier, 2005), pp.65–81.

2   Michael Schwalbe and Douglas Mason-Schrock, 'Identity work as group process' in Barry Markovsky, Michael J. Lovaglia and Robin Simon (eds), *Advances in Group Processes* (Greenwich: JAI Press, 1996), pp.113–47.

3   Patrick J. Carnes, *The Betrayal Bond: Breaking Free of Exploitative Relationships* (Health Communications, Inc., 1997), p.21.

4   Ibid., p.21.

5   Dan Baker et al., 'Youth Chances: Integrated Report', Metro Charity, 2016, https://metrocharity.org.uk/sites/default/files/2017-04/National%20Youth%20Chances%20Intergrated%20Report%202016.pdf

Chapter Three

1   Carlos Cortes, 'A Long Way To Go: Minorities and the Media', Center for Media Literacy, accessed 7 July 2021, www.medialit.org/reading-room/long-way-go-minorities-and-media

2   Cortes, 'A Long Way To Go'.

3   Heather Carey et al., 'Getting In and Getting On: Class, Participation and Job Quality in the UK Creative Industries', Creative Industries Policy and Evidence Centre, University of Edinburgh and Work Advance, August 2020, https://pec.ac.uk/research-reports/getting-in-and-getting-on-class-participation-and-job-quality-in-the-uks-creative-industries

4   'UK Publishing Workforce: Diversity, Inclusion and Belonging', Publishers Association, 11 February 2021, www.publishers.org.uk/publications/diversity-survey-of-the-publishing-workforce-2020/

5   Fred L. Standley and Louis H. Pratt (eds), *Conversations with James Baldwin* (Jackson: University of Mississippi, 1989), p.206.

Chapter Four

1   Michael S. Boroughs, Ross Krawczyk and Joel K. Thompson, 'Body Dysmorphic Disorder Among Diverse Racial/Ethnic and Sexual Orientation Groups: Prevalence Estimates and Associated Factors', *Sex Roles* 63, No. 9–10 (July 2010), 725–737.

2   H.G. Pope, K.A. Phillips and R. Olivardia, *The Adonis Complex: The Secret Crisis of Male Body Image Obsession* (New York: Free Press, 2000).

3   R. Olivardia, 'Body Image and Muscularity' in T.F. Cash and T. Pruzinsky (eds), *Body Image: A Handbook of Theory Research and Clinical Practice* (New York: Guilford Press, 2002), pp.210–218.

4   Joanna Brewis and Gavin Jack, 'Consuming Chavs: The Ambiguous Politics of Gay Chavinism', *Sociology* 44, No. 2 (April 2010), 251–68.

5   Sara B. Kimmel and James R. Mahalik, 'Body Image Concerns of Gay Men: The Roles of Minority Stress and Conformity to Masculine Norms', *Journal of Consulting and Clinical Psychology* 73, No. 6 (2005), 1185–90.

6   'Body Image: How We Think and Feel About Our Bodies', Mental Health Foundation, May 2019, www.mentalhealth.org.uk/publications/body-image-report/sexuality-gender-identity

7   2CV, 'Negative Body Image: Causes, Consequences & Intervention Ideas', Government Equalities Office, August 2019, https://assets.publishing.service.gov.uk/government/uploads/system/uploads/attachment_data/file/952523/Negative_body_image-_causes_consequences__intervention_ideas.pdf

8   'Body image, sexual orientation and gender identity', Mental Health Foundation, www.mentalhealth.org.uk/publications/body-image-report/sexuality-gender-identity

9   2CV, 'Negative Body Image: Causes, Consequences & Intervention Ideas'.
10 Melanie A. Morrison, Todd G. Morrison and Cheryl-Lee Sager, 'Does body satisfaction differ between gay men and lesbian women and heterosexual men and women? A meta-analytic review', *Body Image* 1, No.2 (May 2004), 127–38.
11 L.R. Silberstein, M.E. Mishkind, R.H. Striegel-Moore, C. Timko and J. Rodin, 'Men and their bodies: A comparison of homosexual and heterosexual men', *Psychosom Med* 51, No.3 (May–June 1989), 337–346.

Chapter Five

1   Siri Hustvedt, *A Woman Looking at Men Looking at Women: Essays on Art, Sex, and the Mind* (London: Sceptre, 2017), p.55.
2   Daniel Coleman, Mark S. Kaplan and John T. Casey, 'The Social Nature of Male Suicide: A New Analytic Model', *International Journal of Men's Health* 10, No. 3 (Autumn 2011), 240–52.
3   Jeffrey Weeks, Brian Heaphy and Catherine Donovan, *Same Sex Intimacies: Families of Choice and Other Life Experiments* (London: Routledge, 2001), pp.39–41.
4   'Unlimited Potential: Report of the Commission on Gender Stereotypes in Early Childhood', The Fawcett Society, December 2020, www.fawcettsociety.org.uk/Handlers/Download.ashx?IDMF=17fb0c11-f904-469c-a62e-173583d441c8, p.8.
5   Hustvedt, *A Woman Looking at Men Looking at Women*, p.55.
6   *Unlimited Potential*, p.34.
7   Ibid., p.33.
8   Ibid., p.38.
9   Ibid., p.72.

10 John Tosh, 'Masculinities in an Industrializing Society: Britain, 1800–1914', *Journal of British Studies* 44, No. 2 (April 2005), 338.

11 Alan Sinfield, *The Wilde Century: Effeminacy, Oscar Wilde, and the Queer Moment* (London: Cassell, 1994), pp.25–47, pp.109–26.

12 Daniel Coleman and John Casey, 'The Social Nature of Male Suicide: A New Analytic Model', *International Journal of Men's Health* 10, No.3 (Fall 2011), 240–252.

13 *Unlimited Potential*, pp.71–72.

14 Ibid., p.6.

15 Coleman and Casey, 'The Social Nature of Male Suicide'.

Chapter Six

1 Josh Milton, 'The long, deep, surprisingly versatile history of bottoms: From Ancient Greece to modern misogyny', *PinkNews*, accessed 8 February 2022, www.pinknews.co.uk/2022/02/08/bottoming-history-gay-bottoms/

2 Rictor Norton, 'Mother Clap's Molly House & Deputy Marshall Hitchin: Homosexuality', *The Georgian Underworld: A Study of Criminal Subcultures in Eighteenth-Century England*, 28 January 2012, http://rictornorton.co.uk/gu16.htm

3 Paul Baker, *Polari: The Lost Language of Gay Men* (London: Routledge, 2003) p.73.

4 'Sexual Orientation, UK: 2019', Office for National Statistics, 27 May 2021, www.ons.gov.uk/peoplepopulationandcommunity/culturalidentity/sexuality/bulletins/sexualidentityuk/2019

5 'The Truth About Trans', Stonewall, accessed January 2022, www.stonewall.org.uk/truth-about-trans#trans-people-britain

6 'Figures Reveal LGBTQ+ Venue Numbers Remain Stable for a Second Year', Greater London Authority, 5 July 2019, www.london.gov.uk/press-releases/mayoral/londons-lgbtq-venue-numbers-remain-stable

Chapter Seven

1   Carin Tunåker, 'Flying the flag: Making a difference to homeless LGBTQ youth', Porchlight, www.porchlight.org.uk/downloads/ attachments/Porchlight-lgbt-research.pdf, p.3.

2   Jo Bhandal and Matt Horwood, 'The LGBTQ+ Youth Homelessness Report', AKT, 2021, https://www.akt.org.uk/report, p.3.

Chapter Eight

1   'LGBT+ Experiences in UK Education Improving, New Study Finds', Stonewall, 23 September 2021, www.stonewall.org.uk/about-us/ news/lgbt-experiences-uk-education-improving-new-study-finds

2   David Bell, 'Farm Boys and Wild Men: Rurality, Masculinity, and Homosexuality', *Rural Sociology* 65, No. 4 (December 2000), 547–61; Gretchen Poiner, *The Good Old Rule: Gender and Other Power Relationships in a Rural Community* (Sydney: Sydney University Press, 1990). Sourced from John Scott, Anthony Lyons and Catherine L. MacPhail, 'Desire, Belonging and Absence in Rural Places', *Rural Society: The Journal of Research into Rural and Regional Social Issues in Australia* 24, No. 3 (2015), 219–226.

Chapter Nine

1   Carnes, *The Betrayal Bond*, p.21.

2   Alison Park and Rebecca Rhead, 'British Social Attitudes 30', London: National Centre Social Research, 2013, www.bsa.natcen.ac.uk/ latest-report/british-social-attitudes-30/personal-relationships/ homosexuality.aspx

3   Josh Bradlow, Fay Bartram April Guasp and Vasanti Jadva, 'School
    Report: The experiences of Lesbian, Gay, Bi and Trans Young People
    in Britain's Schools in 2017', Stonewall and University of Cambridge,
    June 2017, www.stonewall.org.uk/system/files/the_school_
    report_2017.pdf, p.4.
4   April Guasp, Gavin Ellison and Tasha Satara, 'The Teacher Report:
    Homophobic Bullying in Britain's Schools in 2014', Stonewall and
    YouGov, January 2015, www.stonewall.org.uk/system/files/teachers_
    report_2014.pdf, p.1.
5   Josh Bradlow, Fay Bartram, April Guasp and Vasanti Jadva, 'School
    Report: The experiences of Lesbian, Gay, Bi and Trans Young People
    in Britain's Schools in 2017', Stonewall and University of Cambridge,
    June 2017, www.stonewall.org.uk/system/files/the_school_
    report_2017.pdf, p.29.
6   Rachael Milsom, 'Growing Up LGBT+:The Impact of School, Home
    and Coronavirus on LGBT+ Young People', Just Like Us, June 2021,
    www.justlikeus.org/single-post/growing-up-lgbt-just-like-us-
    research-report, p.7.
7   Ibid., p.7.
8   Marc Bush, 'Young Minds. Beyond Adversity: Addressing the mental
    health needs of young people who face complexity and adversity in
    their lives', Young Minds, 7 July 2016, www.basw.co.uk/system/files/
    resources/basw_45241-4_0.pdf, p.372.
9   Milsom, *Growing Up LGBT+*, p.45.
10 Ibid., pp.6–7.
11 Bradlow, Bartram, April and Jadva, 'School Report: The experiences of
    Lesbian, Gay, Bi and Trans Young People in Britain's Schools in 2017',
    p.2.

Chapter Ten

1   Pawel Adrjan, 'There's a Gay Wage Gap – And it's Linked
    to Discrimination', *The Conversation*, 29 April 2021, https://theconversation.com/theres-a-gay-wage-gap-and-its-linked-to-discrimination-159956

2   'Just 16% of People in Creative Jobs are from Working Class
    Backgrounds and Those From Privileged Backgrounds More
    Likely to Shape what goes on Stage, Page and Screen', Creative
    Industries Policy and Evidence Centre, 27 August 2020,
    https://pec.ac.uk/news/just-16-of-people-in-creative-jobs-are-
    from-working-class-backgrounds-and-those-from-privileged-
    backgrounds-more-likely-to-land-a-job-experience-autonomy-
    and-progression-and-shape-what-goes-on-stage-page-and-screen

3   Ibid.

4   Carnes, *The Betrayal Bond*, p.14.

5   'New Report into Gay and Bisexual Men's Experience of Sexual
    Violence Published by SurvivorsUK', Survivors UK, accessed 30
    October 2021, www.survivorsuk.org/press-release/new-report-into-
    gay-and-bisexual-mens-experience-of-sexual-violence-published-
    by-survivorsuk/

6   Stuart Haggas, 'Consent and the Gay Community', LGBT Hero,
    accessed 30 October 2021, www.gmfa.org.uk/fs162-consent-and-the-
    gay-community

7   Carol Emslie, Jenna C. Lennox and Lana Ireland, 'The Social
    Context of LGBT People's Drinking in Scotland', Scottish Health
    Action on Alcohol Problems, 15 December 2015, www.shaap.org.uk/
    downloads/86-shaap-glass-report-web-pdf/download.html, p.5.

8   Ibid., p.11.

9   Ibid., p.6.

10 'Chemsex: More than Just Sex and Drugs', Adfam and London Friend,
    2019, https://adfam.org.uk/files/ChemSex_Affected_Others.pdf, p.8.

11 Dima Abdulrahim, Christopher Whiteley, Monty Moncrieff and Owen Bowden-Jones, 'Club Drug Use Among Lesbian, Gay, Bisexual and Trans (LGBT) People', Novel Psychoactive Treatment UK Network, 2016, http://neptune-clinical-guidance.co.uk/wp-content/uploads/2016/02/neptune-club-drug-use-among-lgbt-people.pdf, p.5.

12 'Hidden Figures: LGBT Health Inequalities in the UK', LGBT Foundation, 2020, https://dxfy8lrzbpywr.cloudfront.net/Files/b9398153-0cca-40ea-abeb-f7d7c54d43af/Hidden%2520Figures%2520FULL%2520REPORT%2520Web%2520Version%2520Smaller.pdf, p.33.

13 'Chemsex: More than Just Sex and Drugs', Adfam and London Friend, p.6.

14 Chaka L. Bachmann and Becca Gooch, 'LGBT in Britain – Health Report', Stonewall, 2018, www.stonewall.org.uk/system/files/lgbt_in_britain_health.pdf, p.5.

15 Bachmann and Gooch, 'LGBT in Britain – Health Report', p.5.

16 Carnes, *The Betrayal Bond*, p.22.

17 Ibid., p.22.

18 Elizabeth Saewyc et al., 'School-based Interventions to Reduce Health Disparities Among LGBTQ Youth: Considering the Evidence', McCreary Centre Society & Stigma and Resilience Among Vulnerable Youth Centre, 2016, www.mcs.bc.ca/pdf/considering_the_evidence.pdf, p.17.

Chapter Eleven

1 Rachel, a Hotline Advocate, 'Identifying & Overcoming Trauma Bonds', National Domestic Violence Hotline, accessed 12 November 2021, www.thehotline.org/resources/trauma-bonds-what-are-they-and-how-can-we-overcome-them/

2   Carnes, *The Betrayal Bond*, p.93.
3   Ibid., p.55.
4   'What is trauma bonding', The Chelsea Psychology Clinic, 28 August 2020, www.thechelseapsychologyclinic.com/sex-relationships/what-is-trauma-bonding/
5   Carnes, *The Betrayal Bond*, p.61.
6   Ibid., p.121.
7   Ibid., p.26.
8   'Amendment to the Controlling or Coercive Behaviour Offence', Home Office, updated 31 January 2022, www.gov.uk/government/publications/domestic-abuse-bill-2020-factsheets/amendment-to-the-controlling-or-coercive-behaviour-offence
9   'Statistics on Male Victims of Domestic Abuse', Mankind, accessed 1 April 2022, www.mankind.org.uk/statistics/statistics-on-male-victims-of-domestic-abuse/
10 'Hidden Figures: LGBT Health Inequalities in the UK', LGBT Foundation, 2020, https://dxfy8lrzbpywr.cloudfront.net/Files/b9398153-0cca-40ea-abeb-f7d7c54d43af/Hidden%2520Figures%2520FULL%2520REPORT%2520Web%2520Version%2520Smaller.pdf, p.43.
11 Guasp and Taylor, 'Domestic Abuse: Stonewall Health Briefing', p.6.
12 Catherine Donovan, Rebecca Barnes and Catherine Nixon, 'The Coral Project: Exploring Abusive Behaviours in Lesbian, Gay, Bisexual and/or Transgender Relationships', accessed January 2022, www.pinktherapy.com/portals/0/CourseResources/Coral_Project_Interim_Report_Sept_2014.pdf, p.18.
13 'Evidence from the Male Survivors Partnership', Male Survivors Partnership, 18 February 2021, www.malesurvivor.co.uk/wp-content/uploads/2021/02/Male-Survivors-Partnership-submission-to-2021-VAWG-call-for-evidence.pdf, p.4.
14 Laura Hammond, Maria Ioannou and Martha Fewster, 'Perceptions of male rape and sexual assault in a male sample from the United Kingdom: Barriers to reporting and the impacts of victimization', *Journal of Investigative Psychology and Offender Profiling*, http://eprints.

hud.ac.uk/id/eprint/29241/7/Perceptions%20of%20Male%20Rape%20
and%20Sexual%20Assault.pdf

15 Donovan, Barnes and Nixon, 'The Coral Project', p.8.
16 Ibid., p.25.
17 Bessel van der Kolk, *The Body Keeps the Score* (London: Penguin
Random House, 2014), p.79.
18 van der Kolk, *The Body Keeps the Score*, p.210.

Chapter Twelve

1 van der Kolk, *The Body Keeps the Score*, p.210.
2 Ibid., p.210.
3 Ibid., p.210.
4 Ibid., p.210.
5 Ibid., p.79.
6 Ibid., p.135.

Epilogue

1 Ben Hunte, '"Don't Punish Me For Who I Am": Huge Jump in
Anti-LGBTQ Hate Crime Reports in UK', *VICE*, 11 October 2021, www.
vice.com/en/article/4avkyw/anti-lgbtq-hate-crime-reports-increase-
in-six-years
2 Drinkaware Monitor 2020. Data extracted from following questions:
'Which of the following best describes your sexuality?' 'LGB', n=952
OR 'Is your gender the same as the sex assigned to you at birth? 'No'
n=79.
3 'Hidden Figures: The Impact of the Covid-19 Pandemic on LGBT
Communities', LGBT Foundation, accessed 21 November 2021, https://
lgbt.foundation/coronavirus/hiddenfigures